The Neurodivergent Hormonal Survival Toolkit

A Guide for Neurocomplex People in Peri/Menopause & Their Partners

Expanded Edition

Sarah L. Glasco, Ph.D.

MOD Couple press

Published in the United States of America by Mod Couple Press

A catalog record of this book is on file at the United States Library of Congress.

Cover image by Deagreez c/o Getty Images.

Cover concept and design by Sarah Glasco.

1st edition, May 2026

www.modcouplepress.com

Mod Couple Publishing, LLC

Hillsborough, NC 27278

Praise for The Neurodivergent Hormonal Survival Toolkit

"Finally, a science-backed, no-BS guide to what happens when hormones and neurodivergence collide. Smart, structured, and funny as hell, this toolkit translates complex research into something clear, inclusive, and actually usable. It fills a massive gap in care and does it with heart, humor, and precision."

—Dr. Jen Wolkin (she/her), PhD, MFA, Neuropsychologist & Author of *Quick Calm*

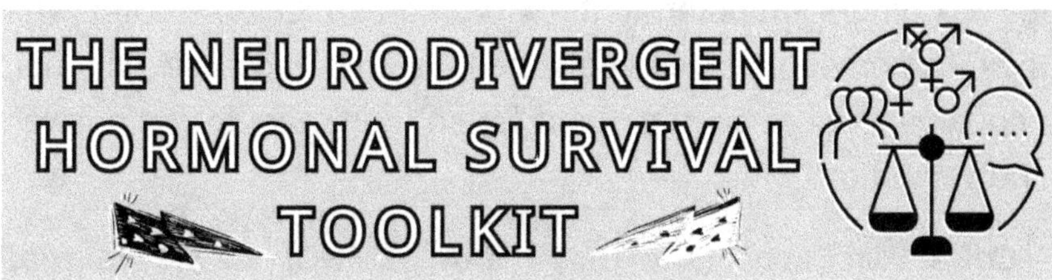

"The Neurodivergent Hormonal Survival Toolkit reads like a love letter to people going through what I affectionately call 'bendy menopause'—we have bendy joints, bendy nervous systems, and bendy genders. Mainstream perimenopause and menopause advice wasn't designed for us, but this book is."

—Vanessa Weiland (she/her), AGPCNP-BC, MSCP, Nurse Practitioner & Founder of Phases Clinic

* * *

"This is not another wellness guide written by someone who took a weekend course and found their purpose. This is a badass former tenured professor and certified menopause consultant who got blindsided by the intersection of neurodivergence and hormones, went balls deep into the research, and built the resource we actually needed. Evidence-backed, accessible by design, and inclusive by conviction."

—Mandi L. Dixon (she/her), LPC, NCC, ADHD and Menopause Therapist & Coach

"This book blew me away! A toolkit like this is hard to find. Sarah perfectly describes the intersections of medical diagnoses, neurotypes, and experiences that many deal with in isolation. More often than not, individuals from our community leave doctors' appointments with more questions than what they came with. I genuinely believe this resource will help people who have been without for so long start to get answers and validation."

—Calial McCarty (she/they), MA, LMHC, CAS, Neuroaffirming Therapist, Founder of The NeuroBloom Center, and author of *Naturally Divergent*

"Forget an algebra book—THIS is the book that needs to be included in every school curriculum (and doctors' offices, community centers, book fairs, Ted Talk, QVC channel—you get the idea.) This is lifesaving, long overdue, yet right on time."

—Elicia Gonzales (she/her), MSW, M.Ed., The Passion Doula

"This book provides a compassionate, evidence-informed guide to understanding the complex interaction between neurodivergence and hormonal change. Sarah Glasco combines research, lived experience, humour and practical tools in a way that makes readers feel seen, validated and empowered. What I particularly appreciate is her ability to explain difficult concepts in an accessible and engaging way, whilst acknowledging the very real challenges many people face when seeking answers and support. An invaluable resource for anyone navigating perimenopause, menopause, and neurodivergence—and for the clinicians, partners and loved ones who want to better understand their experience. This toolkit offers clarity, validation and hope, helping readers understand that they are not broken—they simply deserve better information, support and care."

—Dr. Claire Phipps (she/her), BSC, MBBS, MRCGP, General Practitioner & British Menopause Society accredited Menopause Specialist

"Sarah Glasco is that super-smart friend who always has your back and has done the research so you don't have to. *The Neurodivergent Hormonal Survival Toolkit* is highly readable and packs in a ton of information and heart. It explains why you feel like you're going crazy (you're not), how to ensure you get the help and support you need (you deserve it), and why so much of your life makes sense now (it really does)."

—Dr. Ari Tuckman (he/him), PsyD, MBA, Psychologist & Author of the *ADHD Productivity Manual*

"I love Dr. Glasco's ND Toolkit! It is accessible, by turns deep and hysterical (and I use that term intentionally here), and always human and humane. I absolutely adore the engaging, interactive format, and the Neuro-Hormonal Chaos Decoder chart and affirmation cards are literally life-saving. It is a relief to be so clearly seen and affirmed."

—Lasara Firefox Allen (they/them/Mx.), MSW, author of *Genderqueer Menopause* and Founder of Genderqueer Futures

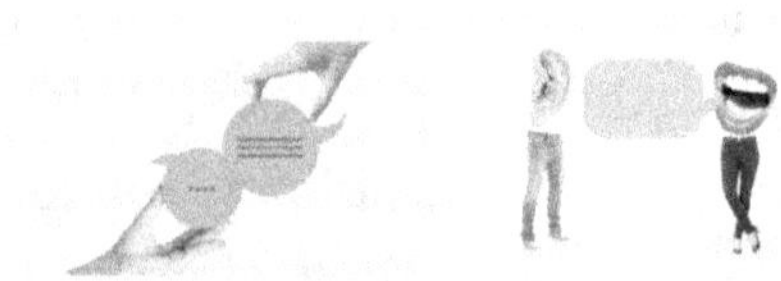

"Are you neurodivergent, perimenopausal, and completely out of spoons? Fear not, Sarah's here with a whole toolkit! This is an absolute must-read. Validating feelings whilst breaking down the science of hormonal hijinx. The book is packed with practical, realistic advice rather than medical monologues and condescending clichés, making it feel like a friend helping you through the chaos. When ADHD and perimenopause collide it can feel like we can't catch a break, but this masterpiece is just the tonic!"

—Laura Mears-Reynolds (she/her), Founder & CEO of ADHDAF+ Charity & Host of the ADHD AF Podcast

* * *

"As a therapist working with neurodivergent adults, I regularly see how disorienting it can be when perimenopause shifts focus, mood, sleep, and daily functioning all at once. It is often misunderstood or brushed off, leaving people trying to piece it together on their own. *The Neurodivergent Hormonal Survival Toolkit* steps into that gap with clarity and direction. Sarah walks readers through symptom identification with her Neuro-Hormonal Chaos Decoder, supports real self-advocacy around those symptoms, and even provides scripts for navigating conversations with medical professionals. She covers how to keep executive functioning moving, offers sleep strategies that go beyond "just go to bed earlier," and emphasizes the importance of community and connection. Grounded in research and built for real life, this is a thoughtful, practical resource I will recommend to my clients."

—Kristin Koliha (she/her), LICSW, Therapist & Founder of Welcome Home ADHD

"As a kid, whenever my school held a book fair, I would make a beeline for the activity books. You know, the ones with stickers and hands-on activities. Sarah's book is a version of that for neurodivergent adults. It is digestible, approachable, fun, and hands-on. What Sarah adds to this book, in particular, is compassion—endless compassion—so much that I found myself pausing and holding back tears. Bravo for putting together this beautiful, heartfelt piece of art for me and for other neurodivergent people who really need it."

—Dr. Gilly Kahn (she/her), PhD, Clinical Psychologist and Author of *Allow Me to Interrupt*

"The Neurodivergent Hormonal Survival Toolkit is a comprehensive research-backed guide for people navigating the confusing collision of hormone changes and executive dysfunction. Packed with practical strategies, relatable insights and a healthy amount of humor, this toolkit will help you understand what's happening in your brain and body without shame or toxic positivity."
—Meredith Carder (she/her), BS Psychology, MBA, ADDCA-trained ADHD Coach & Author of *It All Makes Sense Now*

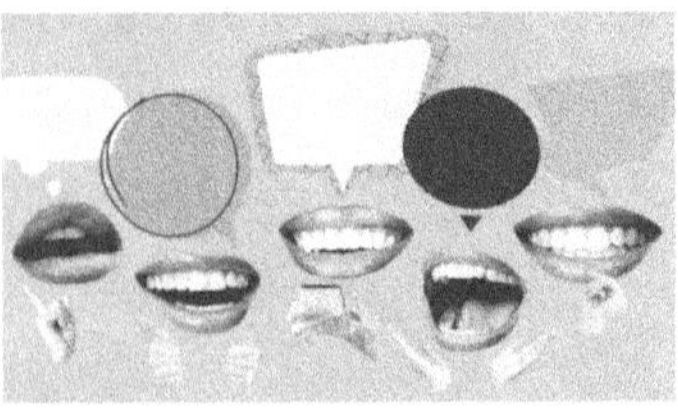

"I really love the way this book breaks down what's actually happening in your body with our hormonal changes. Too many of us end up in perimenopause not knowing what's hit us and this book makes it all make sense. The self-advocacy section is the thing I needed when I was scared to ask for HRT because I didn't know if I'd be taken seriously."

—Paula Hirst (she/her), C.Hpt, Certified ADHD Coach for Women & Founder of ADHD & Alchemy

"In a landscape where both neurodivergence and perimenopause are chronically underrepresented, Sarah brings a refreshing depth of knowledge and genuine care to the conversation. She breaks down a diverse and nuanced subject with remarkable clarity, making complex, life-changing information not only accessible, but deeply meaningful. A vital read for any person navigating these overlapping experiences."
—Julie Murillas, MS, Licensed Professional Counselor

“This is a bold, validating and brilliantly rebellious guide to a space that has been misunderstood, minimised and medicalised for far too long. Sarah Glasco captures the collision of neurodivergence and hormonal change with clarity, humour and political fire, while refusing to leave gender, identity and inclusion at the margins. She translates complex science into something people can actually recognise themselves in, grounding it in applied, lived and embodied politics. This is not just a toolkit. It is a permission slip, a protest sign and a survival guide for those who have been left piecing it all together on their own.”

—Dr. Emma Offord (she/her), PhD, Psychotherapist & Founder of Divergent Life

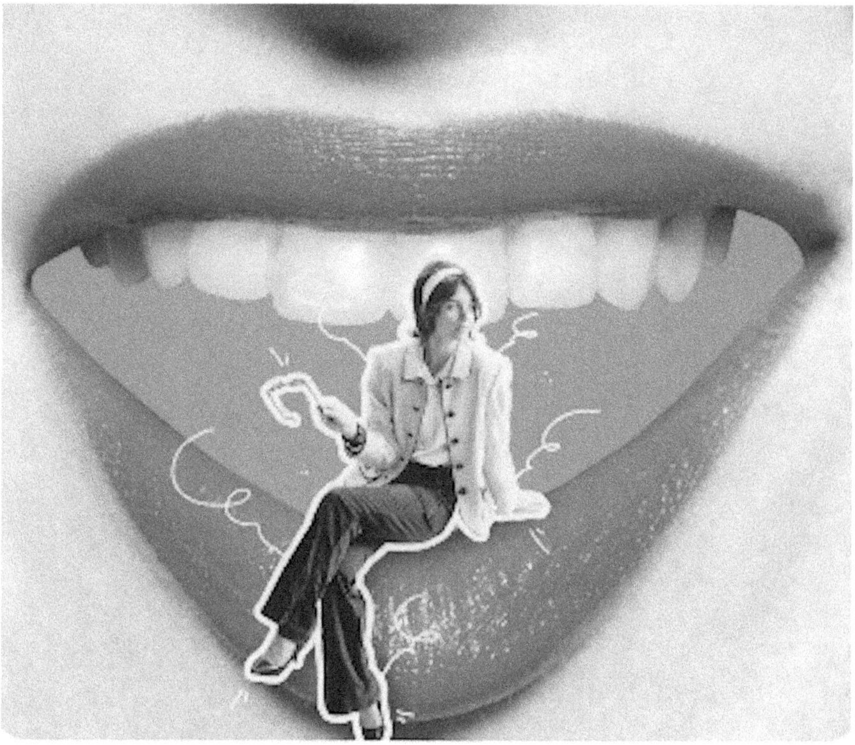

Contents

Medical & Legal Disclaimer

A necessary note before we begin

Hey, Quick Reality Check:

I am not a medical doctor, psychiatrist, nurse practitioner, therapist, pharmacist, or your personal health oracle. I am a lifelong researcher, a lived-experience expert from my cisgender, pansexual-identifying AFAB body perspective, and an unapologetic truth-teller who has done the homework so you don't have to.

While this is for anyone who finds themselves at the crossroads of hormones and neurodivergence—cis, trans, and nonbinary folks alike, partners, clinicians, and all who care for someone in this tangled intersection regardless of race/ethnicity—I acknowledge that despite my aim to be as inclusive as possible, not everyone may be able to see themselves *fully* in these pages. Gender identity, sexual orientation, race, socioeconomic class, diagnosis, and geopolitical culture all shape and impact our experiences, and I don't claim to be an expert in any experience and identity outside my own. I acknowledge my privilege as a white, educated, cis woman and understand that no two ND peri/menopausal odysseys look the same. Take what works for you, and skip what may not.

With this in mind, I've used intentionally more inclusive language throughout and provided a community resource guide at the end of this toolkit where you can find a plethora of perspectives to help you find people, professionals and information that may align more closely with your unique identities. It's not exhaustive by any means, but it's a place to start to enhance your knowledge and grow your own community.

It is NOT a substitute for individualized, professional medical advice, diagnosis, or treatment.

Here's what that means for you:

- Always consult your own healthcare provider before starting, changing, or stopping any medication, hormone therapy, supplement, exercise program, or nutrition plan—especially if you have complex health needs or take other medications.
- This toolkit is for informational, educational, and supportive purposes only. It's designed to help you feel less alone and more prepared, not to replace your doctor, specialist, or therapist.
- If you have questions, concerns, new or worsening symptoms, or a medical emergency, contact your qualified health professional immediately. If you think you're experiencing a medical emergency, dial your country's emergency number (like 911 in the US) right now.

Information provided here—including research summaries, scripts, trackers, cheat sheets, resource links, etc.—is up to date as of publication, but ***medical knowledge and guidelines change FAST.*** *Always verify what's current for your situation.*

I don't provide or claim to provide individual diagnosis, medical care, crisis intervention, or legal advice. I'm not responsible for your health outcomes, choices, or actions resulting from use (or misuse) of this guide.

By purchasing, downloading, or using this toolkit, you acknowledge that you understand and accept these terms. You agree to use this product as intended—as a tool for information and empowerment—and you release and indemnify the creator(s) from any liability, damages, or losses arising from its use.

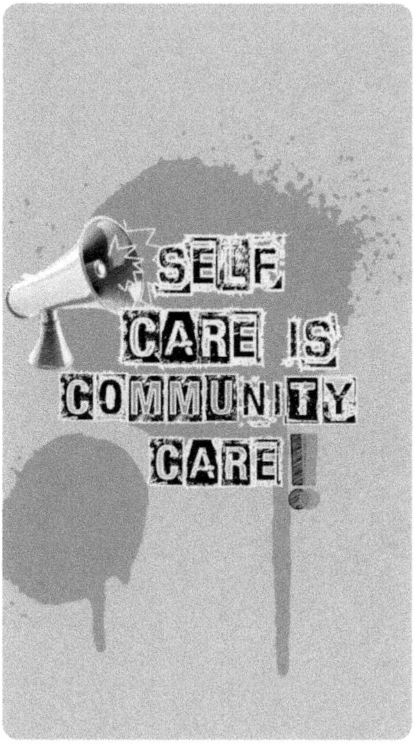

TL;DR: This is a badass, evidence-packed, solidarity-fueled resource, not a medical prescription pad. Trust yourself, question everything, and work with professionals you can trust. You're the expert on your own body—but your health decisions are your responsibility. Stay fierce, stay safe, and never let anyone gaslight you out of getting the care you deserve.

Foreword

I talk to a lot of people about ADHD and perimenopause. On any given day, someone in my neighborhood, email or comments is asking about hormone therapy interactions with stimulant medication, or what brain fog looks like when you're also autistic, or how a trans man with no insurance and no affirming provider is supposed to navigate any of this. I'm a Licensed Professional Counselor, and I specialize in exactly this intersection. And sometimes I still don't have the answer.

That's when I call Sarah.

* * *

What started as a professional connection with Sarah Glasco over a year ago, became something closer to a lifeline. She is my go-to source for the questions that fall through the cracks of the research, which is most of them. The autistic woman in the Australian outback who spent four years trying to get heard before her Hashimoto's diagnosis finally happened. The AuDHD

Black woman who was initially misdiagnosed with Bipolar and had been dismissed in every clinical setting she'd ever walked into. The deaf trans man trying to find menopause care that accommodates his disability and doesn't erase him. These are the people who find me online, who trust me with their most specific and most desperate questions, and who deserve answers that actually account for who they are.

Sarah always has an answer. Whether it's a research article, a connection or just lived experience, she has a tangible solution, and when she doesn't, she will find it. She is the expert for populations that standard menopause literature forgot to include.

The research on cisgender women with ADHD is already limited. I know because that is the majority of people with whom I work. Now add autism, add race, add gender identity, add OCD, add the specific hormonal chaos of perimenopause layered on top of a nervous system that was already working twice as hard just to pass as fine. Add a body that's also been fighting fibromyalgia or POTS or EDS, already exhausted, dismissed, told it's probably just anxiety, and you have a population that has been profoundly, systematically failed and forgotten.

But Sarah didn't forget, and she didn't accept that.

She brought her Ph.D. and all the research methodology, analysis and synthesis skills, and pedagogical tools that that her doctoral degree program provided and helped her refine, her decades of academic rigor as both student, published scholar, and tenured professor, and her own hard-won late diagnosis to this work. She went deep into the research so you wouldn't have to. And she wrote something inclusive by conviction, not by afterthought, because she knows firsthand what it costs when the resource that's supposed to help you doesn't actually see you.

Sarah sees you. You will feel that in this book. She's smart, she's witty, and she's so damn passionate about YOU. I've personally witnessed her step up on a soapbox, tap the mic, and lovingly flail her arms wildly while ranting about the populations of people no one is seeing when it comes to hormonal care in midlife.

This book is for the people who've ever felt like they were too much. The ones who have ever been told their symptoms are anxiety, or stress, or just getting older. It's for the people who masked so well for so long that even they didn't know something was different until everything started falling apart at once. For someone who got their diagnosis at 58, postmenopausal, still grieving, still looking. It's for cis women and gender-expansive people. It's for the partners and families trying to understand what's happening to someone they love and not finding answers anywhere that feel true. This book is for everyone.

It's the resource that should have existed a long time ago. I'm so glad Sarah built it. And I mean that wholeheartedly because I've seen what she does with the questions everyone else can't answer. Nothing about you was ever wrong; you were just never handed the right tools. I'm honored to hand them to you now.

Mandi L. Dixon, MA, LPC, NCC

Allen, Texas

Preface

The great thing about being neurodivergent and an unmasked person in my 50s now is that I don't give a shit what people think of me anymore, and I am not afraid to say what I mean and do what I want. That said, you don't need my permission to skip this preface, but you certainly have it! The rest of the book is in a slightly friendlier format for ND brains that may be easily overwhelmed by big blocks of text like you're seeing here and in the foreword you may (or may not have lol) just read. I may be a bit biased (ok, fine, a lot biased), but you might recognize parts of your story in this preface. There's some compelling shit in here, but you don't need to read it to benefit from this book. So if you're like me and often all over the place, sometimes with the patience of a gnat, yeah, skip on ahead to the intro, or even the first chapter! This part will still be here at the end. But if you're curious and want a bit more in-depth backstory, read on.

Late diagnosis is common in midlife. Many adults reach their forties or fifties before a crisis—burnout at work, relationship struggles, or the sudden collapse of coping skills—prompts them to seek answers. It can be both shocking and oddly comforting to realize that what you labeled as "bad habits" or "laziness" are actually expressions of a neurotype.

The realization that your "quirks" are not moral defects but part of how your brain is wired brings both grief for lost years and relief at no longer blaming yourself.

The first time I can retrospectively now see that peri-menopause was not going to play by the rules (hindsight can be so cruel and hilarious), I was in my early 40s. I sat in my doctor's office explaining a surge of symptoms that seemed to appear out of nowhere. My hands trembled—from nerves, because going to the doctor knowing they're going to check my blood pressure always gives me anxiety despite my history of healthy blood pressure—but also the mix of exhaustion and adrenaline that had been a new amped-up extension of my already fatigue-ridden norm. I described memory lapses, constant irritation at every sound, and a growing sense of mental fog. The doctor smiled and said, "That's just stress and fatigue. It happens to everyone." I remember asking her if it could be pre-menopause (because I don't think the word peri-menopause was part of my vocabulary yet). I explained that I had started experiencing pretty intense night sweats around age 39/40, but that I had done some research and had started taking Black Cohosh for them. Of course, hearing about anything natural/herbal coupled with the fact that I had consulted Dr. Google instead of her was met with a smirk and perceived tinge of dismissal.

Nevertheless, she did a menopause blood panel that day, which came back "normal," and therefore, she told me, I was nowhere near menopause. I was "fine." The problem was, I was not fine.

In fact, I was a closet basket-case just triaging my own mental health literally on a minute-by-minute basis.

When I went back for a follow-up a few months later, I broke down completely. To my doctor's credit, she took it very seriously and spent 90 minutes with me for an appointment that was supposed to last 30 minutes (all apologies to the poor souls who had appointments after me and were left waiting what may have become a rage-induced, excessive amount of time ...). I could no longer mask how unwell I was. I sobbed the entire time while attempting to explain that I felt like something was very wrong with me mentally because none of the medications she had prescribed to me prior had ultimately helped.

She asked me about my periods, how long they were, how heavy the flow was, length of time between each cycle, etc. But I knew this wasn't just a simple hormonal phase—it was a puzzling experience no one seemed willing to help me untangle. After all, I had a PhD, a "prestigious" demanding job, what seemed like a very stable family life. On paper, I had it all. (I was also addicted to running, so this undoubtedly helped my mental health enough to keep my flying under the radar. There's no way someone like me could have ADHD ... Insert eye roll here, but hey, again, we didn't know what we didn't know.)

After 90 minutes with her that day, I walked out with a prescription for Wellbutrin, and spent the next 10 years on it. While it did help me (and I would later learn that it is sometimes prescribed off-label for ADHD), it still didn't adequately address the root problems: yet-to-be-discovered ADHD, OCD, dyslexia (I know, right?!), hypermobility, definite autistic traits (though no formal diagnosis on that one), and fluctuating/declining estrogen due to perimenopause—which profoundly affects your entire body and brain, and hence, both your mental and physical health. Thus, Wellbutrin could only do so much to improve my wellbeing.

Let me quickly say this: I trust and respect my doctor. This is not meant as a slight to her or any other medical provider. OK, fine, that's technically a lie. It is a slight to the shit providers out there whose egos are too big for their own good, the ones who don't listen, and minimize or even dismiss your pain and suffering as normal, acceptable, and even possibly your own fault or in your head. As with any service provider in life, there are good ones, and yes, there are some really bad ones out there. My personal physician is not one of the bad ones.

Primary care providers don't always have time to become experts on neurodivergence and hormonal health, let alone the chaotic collision of both. Like me, my doctor simply didn't know what she didn't know, and as someone my age, to her credit, she has learned a lot about neurodivergence and peri/menopause since then. It's not abnormal for primary care physicians to not know much about your ADHD or your kid's autism or perimenopause or the fact that your pronouns are now they/them and you're experiencing gender dysmorphia. They are called GPs for a reason. GP stands for general practitioner, but let's not underestimate the pressure of being expected to know a little bit about literally everything. I don't take for granted the education that medical providers have. Just because GPs aren't specialists per se, it would be incorrect to characterize them as "jack of all trades, master of none." They know a lot. But it is unreasonable to expect them to know everything. That's why they refer to specialists when problems arise that are outside their scope of practice or field of expertise. It's how they proceed, however, once you hand over new facts and useful information to them that matters most.

Never underestimate the importance and necessity of respect. Never be afraid of demanding the respect you deserve.

All that to say, if you've ever left an appointment feeling any degree of dismissal, no matter how slight, feeling led to believe that you were exaggerating your symptoms, or left wondering why typical advice fails you, this book will make you feel seen. Here, your confusion is real, and your experience is valid. I believe you.

Now, fast forward to years later. I had been on Wellbutrin for six years or so at this point. I was standing in my kitchen, holding a list of things I needed to do, the COVID pandemic was raging, I was teaching remotely, and having my daughter (also undiagnosed AuDHD and OCD at the time and struggling mightily, but that's another story) home to do school Online was so freaking hard, and my mind went blank. Completely blank. Not a gentle "Oh, what was I doing?" but a deep, bone-shaking void kind of blank. My heart pounded. I could not remember why I had opened the fridge or where I had put the bag of groceries I had just brought into the house a few minutes prior. My hands were shaking, and the noise from the refrigerator felt louder than a freight train. I was having another now familiar panic attack, but this one felt different. I used my normal coping strategies of stopping what I was doing to go outside and get fresh air and to call a "safe" friend or talk to my partner—people I trusted and who knew about my panic attacks and how to help me when they were occurring—but I was still unsettled.

I took a few more minutes and managed to get my blood pressure and pulse stabilized, and so I went back inside and carried on making dinner. But the emotional dysregulation I was still experiencing felt visceral. Primal. Unhinged. What happened next was mortifying to me at the time. Looking back, well ... it's still mortifying on some level, but it all makes sense now. Nevertheless, at the time, I was horrified. Embarrassed. And deeply troubled.

It was late spring 2020. We had a nice family dinner planned that evening with my kids—my son, almost 19, and my daughter who was 14 at the time—and I completely broke down right as we began to eat. I was sobbing, nay, ugly-cry-gasping-for-air, and apologizing to my family, reassuring them that I was ok, that I had just had a really hard week at work, and that I didn't know why I was crying so much, but that I couldn't control it. Tears were literally falling onto my plate of pasta. I could tell that my kids were so confused. The roles were suddenly reversed. I was always the one doing everything, handling everything. Taking care of everyone. But out of the blue, I was a fucking wreck, and it was more complex than I would have ever imagined. They wanted to help, but they weren't sure what to do. I tried to laugh through my sobbing to throw in my trademark self-deprecating humor, to offer some levity in what was realistically a total shit show. I succeeded somewhat: they managed some forced half-smiles and laughs, but there was no hiding behind a mask that evening. Something was clearly wrong, and they knew it.

I felt terrible. I felt like I had ruined the dinner. The moment. The evening. In retrospect, it was so dramatic that there really was no turning it around. The air was irrevocably awkward; but then, my son—an AuDHDer himself who has his own sensory issues and doesn't like to be touched—did something shocking: he stood up from the table and asked me if I needed a hug. My typical response might have been, "no, it's ok. I appreciate it. I'm ok," because I was always the one making sure everyone else was ok, always minimizing my pain. Instead, I laugh-cry-sighed with relief and replied, "Actually, yes. Yes, I do." I know we held each other for at least six seconds, but I can't remember if it was much longer than that. (Not to go off on an ADHD tangent here, but if you're not up on the research, hugs ... if you're receptive to/of them, because I feel like that might matter ... lasting six seconds or more trigger the brain to start releasing oxytocin. However, to experience a significant surge of this hormone—which actively lowers cortisol and literally has the power to reduce pain—experts recommend hugs of at least 20 seconds for more potential dopamine activation. Google it! That shit's real.) Regardless, he either somehow instinctively understood what I needed most in that moment or he had the wisdom to simply understand that even if he couldn't fix me, he could try and soothe me, and I was grateful for his effort.

I was 48, a mother, a professor, and a woman who had spent her life forcing her brain to fit into other people's boxes. That night, I wondered if I was losing my mind. Again. Feeling like an unfixable hot mess had really begun to be the norm for me as someone who had been prescribed a plethora of anti-depressants and medications for insomnia that never ultimately solved any of my "problems" throughout my 30s and 40s.

Well, DUH, yeah, I was absolutely perimenopausal—while continuing to live with undiagnosed ADHD, OCD, and dyslexia et al. on top of my queerness that I had never truly publicly disclosed. My partner (who is a bisexual cis man) knows I am pansexual as do close friends, but it's not something I had discussed much with anyone. That evening, I felt so very small and incredibly alone. Don't get me wrong: the hug from my son was absolute medicine in the moment. A salve for my withered soul. But like everything else that had been offered to me, it was triage. Like putting a bandaid on an enormous gash that needed stitches and antibiotics. A temporary remedy.

If you have ever found yourself overwhelmed by both your brain and your body, this book is for you. We are told that menopause is "just a phase" or that it is "natural"—as if that makes it any easier. When you add multi-layered neurodivergence to the mix, you face a storm that most people do not see or understand. The medical world rarely talks about what happens when sensory overload, hormonal chaos, and executive dysfunction collide. Too often, we are dismissed, misdiagnosed, or told to "just relax." There is a gap between what we need and what we get. That gap is wide, and it is lonely.

And that is partly why I wrote this book, because I know what it feels like to live in that gap. But that gap isn't the only one ...

Introduction

Recent Research, Intersectionality, and Inclusion: Why Neurodivergent Menopause Still Feels Like Uncharted Territory

Inclusive in Theory, Binary in Practice: Beyond "Female ADHD" & Why Research on Hormones and Neurodivergence Must Name Gender Diversity: A response to a position paper on the current research on ADHD in particular + hormones and its systemic gaps.

Kooij et al.'s 2025 position paper is important, overdue, and in many ways genuinely useful. It clearly argues that ADHD in girls and women has been "under-recognised and under-researched," and it highlights how puberty, menstrual cycling, pregnancy, and menopause can shape ADHD symptoms, mood, and executive functioning across the lifespan. The authors also explicitly state that the aim is to better understand ADHD in "people assigned female at birth" and acknowledge "non-binary individuals, and transgender men."

And yet this is exactly where the paper starts arguing with itself.

If the stated aim is to understand ADHD in people assigned female at birth, then continuing to frame the conversation primarily through the language of "female," "girls," and "women" is not fully inclusive. It is better than silence, yes, but it still leaves a structural gap. Many trans men, nonbinary people, and other gender-expansive AFAB individuals also live through puberty, menstruation, pregnancy, surgical menopause, perimenopause, and menopause-related hormonal shifts that can affect attention, mood, cognition, and treatment response. When those realities are acknowledged in passing but not carried through the title, framing, and terminology, inclusion starts to look more decorative than structural.

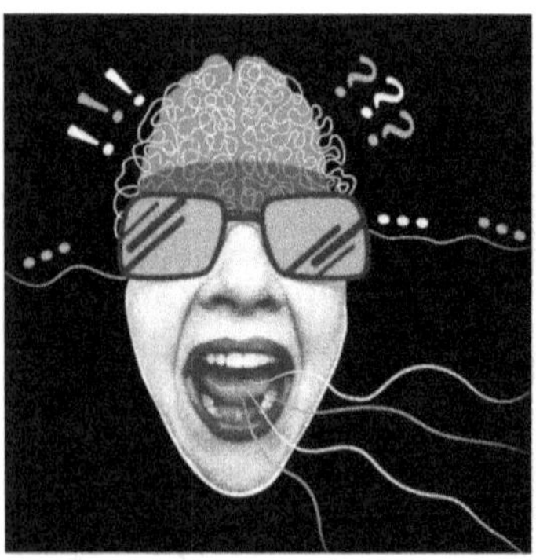

That gap matters even more because this is not some tiny niche population hidden in the margins of clinical care. Anecdotally, many clinicians and community members have noticed substantial overlap between neurodivergence and queer or gender-diverse populations for years. The research now backs that up. Warrier et al. (2020), using five large datasets, found that transgender and gender-diverse individuals had elevated rates of autism diagnosis, autistic traits, and related neurodevelopmental and psychiatric conditions, including ADHD. A separate review by Goetz et al. concluded that prior work suggests increased ADHD prevalence among transgender and gender-diverse individuals.

Research on autism and sexual orientation also shows that autistic people are more likely to report non-heterosexual orientations than non-autistic peers. In other words, inclusive language here is not a side issue. It is central to scientific accuracy.

The paper's conclusion actually sharpens this critique, because the authors call for "Longitudinal inclusive cohort studies that track individuals with ADHD of different genders across life stages" and for "sex and gender-sensitive tools." Good. They should. But that makes the persistent binary framing even harder to ignore. If the future research agenda is meant to be inclusive across genders, then the publication language should reflect that now, not later.

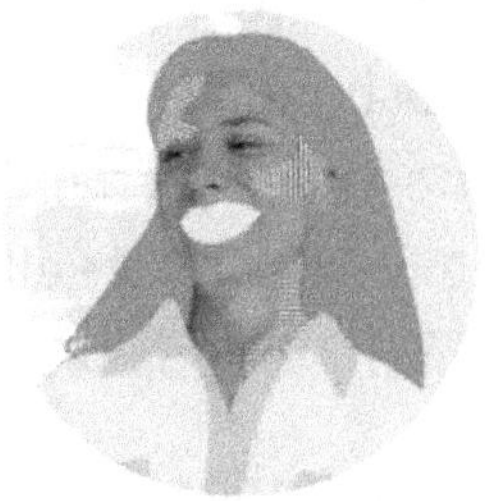

A relatively simple shift would go a long way: when the topic is ovarian hormones, menstruation, reproductive transitions, or menopause-related physiology, use **AFAB** or **people assigned female at birth** rather than using "female" as a catch-all. Better still, future studies could simply say **people born with ovarian systems** and should explicitly name **cisgender girls and women, trans men, nonbinary people, and other gender-expansive AFAB individuals** in their research agendas, recruitment, reporting, and publication language. That is not semantic fussiness. It is the difference between saying inclusion matters and building it into the science.

This paper is still progress. But progress that acknowledges exclusion while continuing to reproduce binary language is incomplete progress. If ADHD research truly wants to become more equitable, then its language, samples, and frameworks need to reflect the full range of people whose lives are shaped by these hormonal and neurodevelopmental realities—not just the people medicine has historically found easiest to name. And that matters.

Equity and accessibility matter.

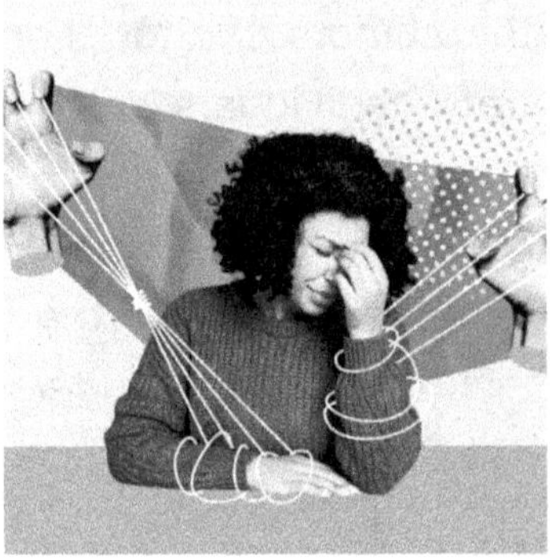

What This Means for You

If you're reading this book, you are already part of the solution. You're refusing to accept invisibility, dismissal, or one-size-fits-all care. The time for hand-waving and gaslighting is over. *Everyone* deserves research, resources, and real-world support that actually work for all neurodivergent folks who will go through peri/menopause, regardless of gender identity.

The authors conclude: "By prioritising hormonal and inflammatory pathways and adopting inclusive, lifespan-focused research designs, the field can advance towards more effective, gender-sensitive ADHD care;" however, if this so-called "gender-sensitive" care is rooted in a gender binary, it's ultimately neither sensitive nor inclusive.

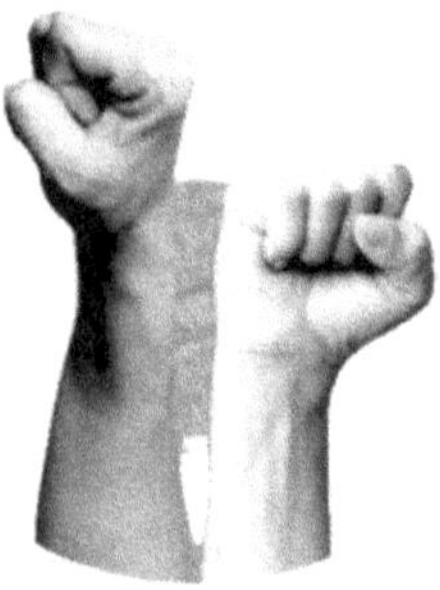

It's time to build a genuinely inclusive future that understands that gender is a cultural construct — one where all stories matter and rebellious acts of self-advocacy are rooted in community care.

* * *

References:

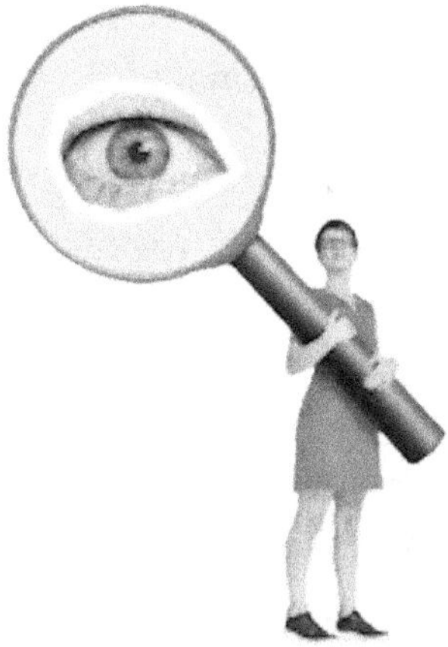

Kooij, J. J. S., de Jong, M., Agnew-Blais, J., et al. (2025). Research advances and future directions in female ADHD: the lifelong interplay of hormonal fluctuations with mood, cognition, and disease. *Frontiers in Global Women's Health*, 6, 1613628.

Dewinter, J., De Graaf, H., & Begeer, S. (2017). Sexual orientation in autism spectrum disorder. *Autism Research, 10* (5), 930–941.

Goetz, T. G., Adams, N. J., Schiwe, T., et al. (2024). The transgender and gender diverse and attention deficit hyperactivity disorder nexus: A systematic review. *Journal of Gay & Lesbian Mental Health*. Advance online publication.

Warrier, V., Greenberg, D. M., Weir, E., et al. (2020). Elevated rates of autism, other neurodevelopmental and psychiatric diagnoses, and autistic traits in transgender and gender-diverse individuals. *Nature Communications, 11*, 3959.

Recommended Reads

Genderqueer Menopause: Navigating menopause for trans, gender-nonconforming, genderfluid, and other queer-bodied folx by Lasara Firefox Allen (North Atlantic Books, 2026)

Menopause: The intersection of race, neurodivergence, and mental health by Amalka (in *Medium*, October 22, 2025)

OK. Thanks for bearing with me. I had to make my point. Most of you probably have no idea who I am, so allow me to introduce myself a bit more formally, informally, professionally, albeit unprofessionally ...

I'm Sarah Glasco (she/her) — ex-professor, author, educator, unapologetic research nerd, podcast host, and a late-diagnosed neurodivergent pansexual person who's spent a lifetime navigating invisible mazes.

I've lived through the whiplash of perimenopause and menopause and spent years in the trenches of academia, advocacy, and radical self-discovery.

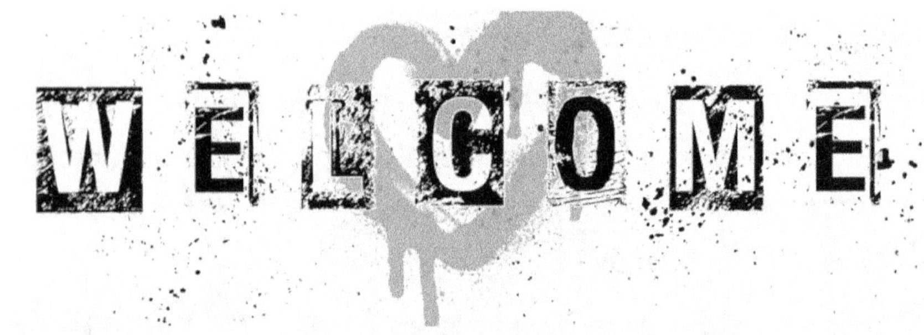

In fact, I'm still doing it. Like you, I've had my share of dismissive doctors, baffling symptoms, and those “am I the only one?” moments.

At 51, I was diagnosed with ADHD, OCD, and dyslexia. By then I'd already raised two neurodivergent kids, earned a PhD, gotten tenure, published a book, left a 20+ years marriage, and survived a decades-long performance of normalcy that nearly killed me.

People called me brilliant. A visionary. A rock star.

But I wasn't thriving.

I was rationing energy, faking functionality, and frankly wondering every day when it would finally all fall apart.

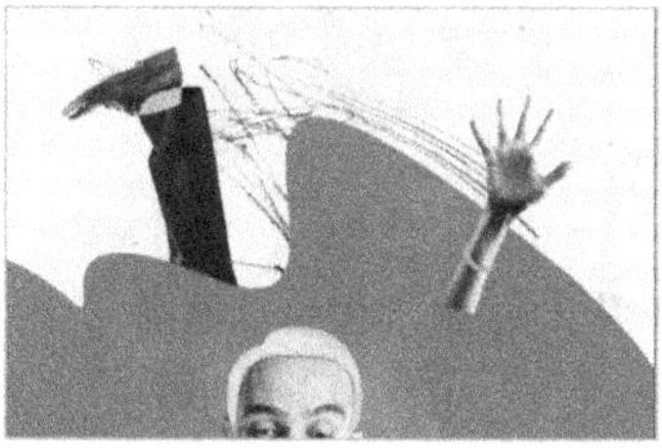

What no one saw, what even I couldn't name, was the cost of holding it all together without ever knowing why everything felt so damn hard.

I masked my burnout with productivity. I buried my trauma under achievement. I used my job as proof that I was "fine."

But I wasn't.

And in January 2023, after one rare, full night of sleep, I woke up with a kind of indignant clarity I hadn't felt in years. I remember pacing the house, ranting to my partner, *"Is this what* NORMAL *people get to feel like all the time?"*

Unbeknownst to me, I was on the cusp of menopause (six months out from my last period) with a multitude of undiagnosed neurobiological conditions, and I was clueless about it all.

I'd planned to go to work that day.

Instead, I set up a meeting with my department chair and quit.

I got my diagnoses eight months later. Nine months later, my dad died. I simultaneously grieved the perceived loss of an entire life spent not fitting in and feeling broken, the loss of my father (and really, both parents since my mom had passed away in 2020), and my chance to be a better, more neuroaffirming parent to my kids while they were still young, among so many other things.

I was angry and sad and frustrated.

- How could I have not known?
- How could others have not suspected?
- Why did I myself not even consider that perimenopause was raging after 6 months without a period?

HOW DID ANY OF THIS GO UNDETECTED?!

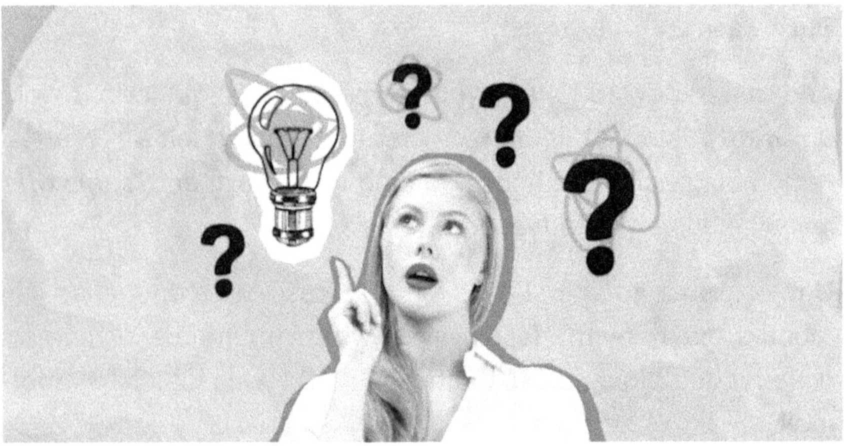

☒ I knew nothing about hormones and neurotransmitters.

☒ I knew nothing about the implications and real life disruptive consequences of estrogen decline.

☒ I had never heard of progesterone lol, ok maybe, but barely.

☒ I did not realize that testosterone was a human hormone, not a uniquely male hormone.

☒ I had no clue what dopamine did.

☒ I didn't even realize that the anti-depressant I had been on for 8 years at that point (Wellbutrin) was an NDRI (a norepinephrine dopamine reuptake inhibitor ... I thought it was an SSRI, just like all the others I had been prescribed in years past with little success.)

✔ I did know that serotonin was known as the "happy hormone."

✔ I knew that cortisol was a stress hormone, and ...

✔ I knew that running released a shit ton of endorphins for me.

Those *obvious* signs—soaked sheets, hot flashes, rage moshing into the void—they're just Act 1 of the Hormonal Shit Storm.

The earliest physical symptoms are really red flags for what's already happening *invisibly*:

- bone loss
- subtle hair loss
- joint pain
- cognitive impairment
- chronic inflammation running riot through your body as estrogen declines

And when estrogen drops? Dopamine follows.

That's why peri/menopause hits neurodivergent people harder — because our wiring was already hustling for scraps, and now the system's on fire.

There's a lot of grief. But the more I began to learn about neurodivergence and menopause individually + collectively, the more I felt a cathartic sense of relief. I now understand the reasons why I think the way I think and feel the way I feel.

➡ My brain is literally wired differently due to a neurobiological condition I was born with (thanks, ADHD, and all the co-morbidities that accompany mine ... I'm talking to you, OCD, Dyslexia, auditory processing issues, sensory sensitivities, and hypermobility), and

➡ My body and brain were in a biochemical civil war with deep neurological impacts AKA perimenopause.

The collision of these two is complete hormonal havoc. Understand this clearly: Treatment for neurobiological conditions and neurological chemical imbalances is preventative care. Menopause care is preventative care.

For many folks, if they don't already know they're neurodivergent, this hormonal hellscape is what finally reveals it—because masking gets harder when your brain and body are both in revolt.

It's important to understand that the definition of neurodivergence is not just academic; it determines who gets seen, supported, and understood. Narrow definitions leave out huge numbers of people who need help during menopause but do not fit into neat diagnostic categories. If you have ever looked for resources and found only discussions of autism or ADHD, never seeing mention of dyspraxia, dyslexia, dyscalculia, hypermobility and Ehlers-Danlos syndromes (EDS), Tourette's, or OCD, CPTSD, Bipolar, and so on, you know how isolating this can feel.

The neurodivergent umbrella is expansive. Recognizing the spectrum means acknowledging the full range of experiences and honoring the complexity of every reader's story. It calls for language that is strengths-based—a refusal to reduce anyone to a checklist of symptoms or a stereotype. Thus, the choice of "neurocomplex" in the book subtitle.

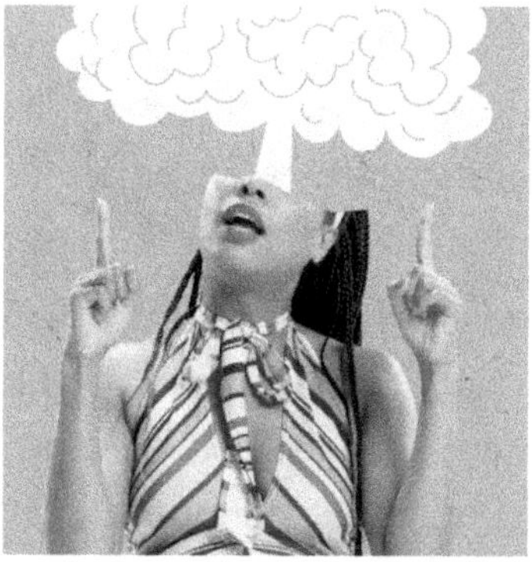

While this book can't constantly allude to or even name every neurotype and condition (let alone discuss them in detail) and admittedly does lean heavily on ADHD/Autism, know that this is merely a point of departure for more profound conversations you can begin initiating with your medical providers and loved ones in order to get the care you deserve. You are not broken. You are neurodivergent, and you deserve nuanced care for what may well be the complexity of your individual ND conditions.

Black/Brown/Indigenous Communities + Gender Diversity, and the Exclusion that Persists

The *gap in research* on ***cisgender women with ADHD and/or Autism*** is jarring enough.

The impact of hormones on ***neurodivergent cis women and girls***? Emerging in recent years, but still very sparse when compared to boys with ADHD and Autism and men's hormonal health.

Studies centering ***gender diverse folks and BIPOC in menopause*** alone? Neglected. Throw in the ***intersection of the myriad of neurodivergences in marginalized populations***? Practically nonexistent.

Indeed, most of the resources and conversations exclude gender-expansive populations and still frame peri/menopause in terms of a gender binary that addresses only cis women, leaving out millions of ***trans and nonbinary people*** who will also go through peri/menopause. Not withstanding that there is research that highlights higher rates of neurodivergence among LGBTQIA+ and gender diverse populations, for many of us, what happens when a complex neurodivergent mind (that perhaps includes OCD like mine, and a bendy body with hypermobility and thus connective tissue issues like mine, for example) collides with rapidly changing hormones is also part of the big picture and needs to be acknowledged as interconnected.

We must continue to name that most of the participants in the published studies emerging on both menopause and neurodivergence individually and collectively are primarily cisgender, heterosexual, *white* women (Lewis Johnson, T. Et al., 2024).

Systemic racism is alive and thriving in science and the funding for research on historically marginalized populations.

Make no mistake: this gap isn't theoretical. It is structural, and it matters. It shapes life in subtle but profound ways. Diagnostic tools, built on white, male norms, often erase subtle differences in neurodivergence seen in people of color, leading to delayed diagnosis, missed treatment, and real harm. Black neurodivergent women, in particular, are far more likely to have their pain dismissed or symptoms attributed to "stress" or "attitude," rather than being taken seriously.

The overlap between menopause symptoms and neurodivergent traits creates confusion and heightens distress, but all of this is amplified if you're being excluded from the conversations and funded studies. This reality needs to be stated loudly, and it needs to change. More on this in the Afterword.

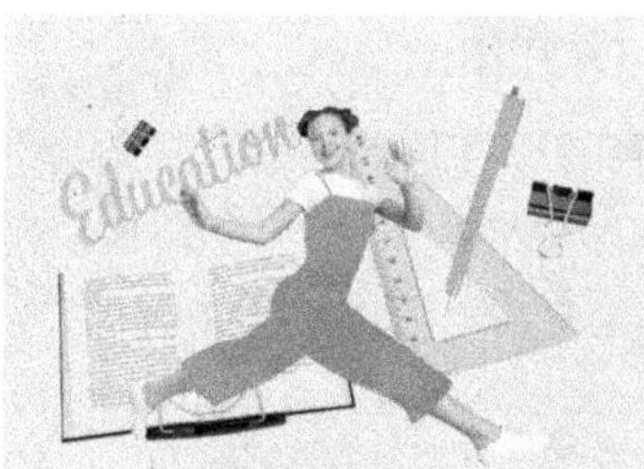

I've made it my mission and life's work now to advocate for, educate, and inform neurodivergent humans and their partners and chosen families because menopause is not a gendered issue.

It's a global healthcare crisis that affects everyone, and inclusivity matters.

I don't want anyone coming up behind me to be ambushed by menopause and late-diagnosed neurodivergence like I was, and no one should be left behind in these conversations and research studies due to race, ethnicity, socioeconomic status, and gender identity. Menopause doesn't just happen to cis white women, and the sooner we understand that **inclusive menopause care is gender-affirming care and that gender-affirming care benefits EVERYONE,** the more just and healthy we will all be.

This toolkit is the resource I wish I'd had when everything started to unravel—and then finally made sense.

Sarah L. Glasco, Ph.D.

As a career academic and former tenured professor who researched, published, and presented scholarly literature regularly, I have the skills and the passion to cull through the research on neurodivergence and midlife hormonal fluctuations so you don't have to. I also taught Women's, Gender & Sexualities Studies courses and am currently training to be an IPHM (International Practitioners of Holistic Medicine) accredited certified menopause doula/coach. And I completed an IAOTH (Int'l Association of Therapists) accredited certification in gender-affirming menopause care in April 2026 and have begun to offer one-time menopause care consultations to help folks who need extra support strategize their steps in developing a path to the nuanced and individualized treatment they deserve.

This book includes evidence-backed scholarship from a cross-section of the most cutting-edge and up-to-date studies available, condensed and curated into this concise and user-friendly guide with accessibility at the forefront of my mind always. I draw on current research from psychiatry, neurology, endocrinology, and the lived experience of the neurodivergent community.

It's a neurodivergent hormonal survival toolkit in accessible narrative form, and it's for me, you, for all of us. This book has heart, but it is, above all, practical. It is designed for you to use in real time—at home, at work, in relationships, in your doctor's office—and not even in any specific order.

Inclusivity is not a footnote here; it is the fucking foundation. It's built for anyone who finds themselves at the crossroads of hormones and neurodivergence—AFAB, cis, trans, nonbinary folks, partners, clinicians, and all who care for or about someone in this precarious intersection. Gender, race, class, diagnosis, and culture shape our experiences, and no two ND peri/menopausal odysseys look the same.

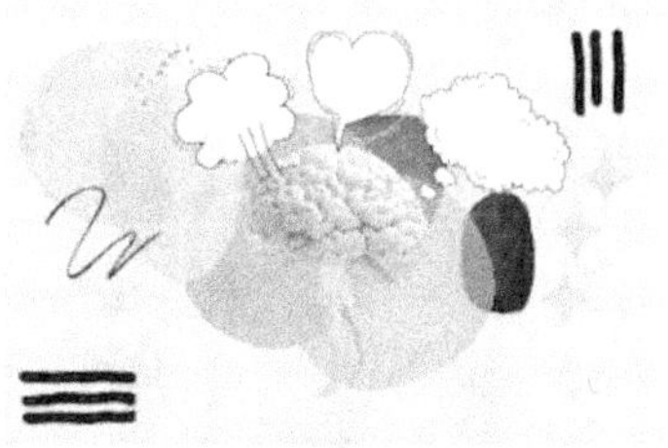

This book does not assume that one size fits all. I know it doesn't. It was written for brains that zig when others zag. It has made efforts to honor sensory differences, emotional intensity, and the many ways our experiences are both unique and shared. Neurodivergent people process information differently, and as a dyslexic person who has struggled significantly with reading comprehension and processing delays, the format and presentation of the information here is important to me.

What you'll see:

- Intentional smaller chunks of text
- A dyslexia-friendly sans-serif font
- Larger fonts used intermittently
- Bullet points
- A variety of formatting and layouts
- Images throughout

➡ Images paired with text help neurodivergent brains by reducing cognitive load, enhancing memory retention, and improving comprehension.

➡ Visuals may also act as anchors to decode information faster, bridging gaps in working memory, particularly for individuals with dyslexia or ADHD.

If you're diagnosed, self-identified, or just "wondering," cisgender, queer, trans or nonbinary, Black, white, Asian, Indigenous, Latinx, you belong here, no matter your age, gender identity, gender

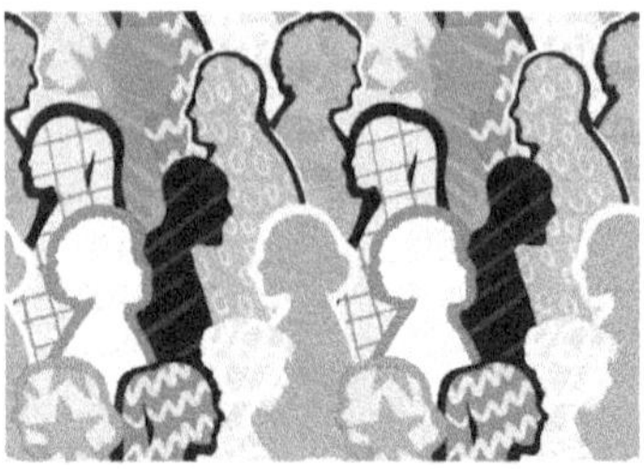

expression, sexual orientation, race, ethnicity, neurotype or star sign.

Read that again: you belong here.

What you'll find inside:

1. Science-backed, no-bullshit explanations of what's happening in your body and brain
2. Validation, humor, and real talk from someone who's been through it
3. Actionable tools, charts, affirmations, and scripts for every step of the journey
4. Community resources and podcast links for when you need a dose of "same here" solidarity

How to use this toolkit:

- *Move through each chapter at your own pace.*
- *Start with whatever feels most urgent — or just flip to a resource and use it as needed.*
- *This is not a course you have to "finish" to benefit.*
- *Each chapter stands alone, but together, they form a roadmap for navigating the chaos with more clarity, self-compassion, and community.*

You are not too much, too late, or too complicated.

You are exactly where you need to be — and you are never alone here. You've taken a substantial step toward understanding and advocating for yourself by investing in this resource.

Ultimately, my hope is that you will finish this book feeling part of something bigger than yourself.

Courage is not about never feeling fear or doubt. It is about moving forward even when the way is unclear. You belong here. Whether you are neurodivergent, peri/menopausal, a partner, or a provider, you are not alone. This book is a call to courage and belonging—for me, for you, for all of us who refuse to disappear into the margins. It might sound cliché, but let's find our way, together. Things are easier, and we are better *together.*

You're ready to feel empowered. Now let's get into the real work — chapter by chapter.

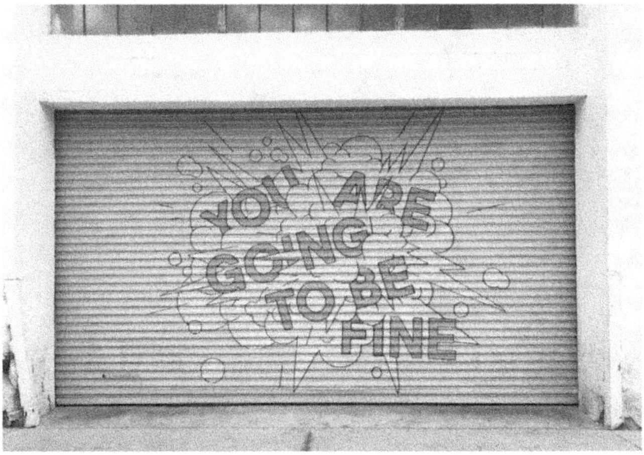

If you ever feel lost, overwhelmed, or alone, refer back to the included glossary or take a break and listen to the podcast. We're in this together.

With empathy, science, and more than a little punk spirit,

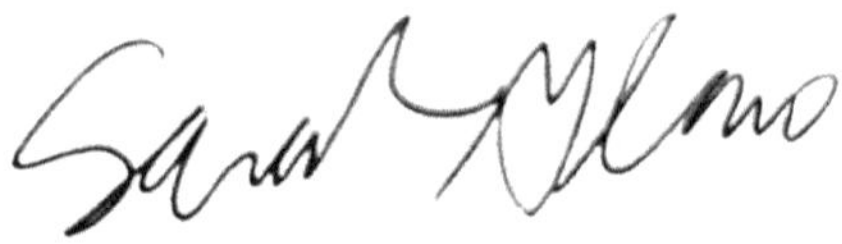

Sarah L. Glasco, Ph.D. (she/her/hers)

Chapter 1

Decode & Validate Your Experience

Theme: Clarity

Goal: Help you immediately recognize the neurodivergent-specific signs of perimenopause and menopause—and understand you're not alone, you don't need fixing, and you're NOT imagining things.

* * *

You're not broken.
You're navigating the intense intersection of hormonal upheaval and neurodivergence. This is your science-backed guide to clarity.

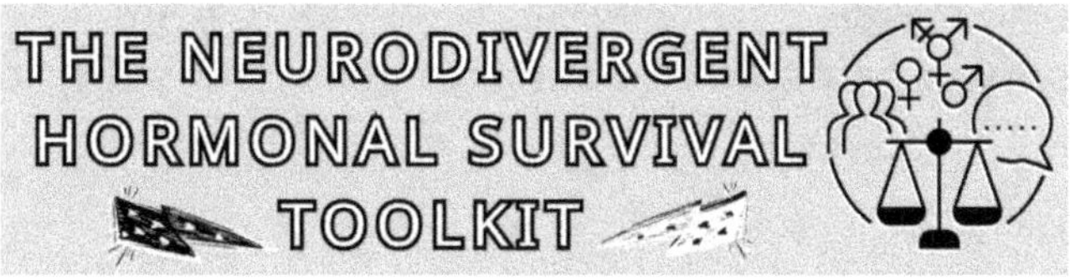

Welcome & Why This Matters More Than Ever

You've heard it all before.

You've been told "it's just stress," "you're fine," "that's normal," or my personal favorite — "you're too young for that."

Hormonal fluctuations—especially during perimenopause and menopause—can dramatically amplify ADHD and autistic traits, making life feel chaotic.

You keep wondering: **WTF Is Happening to Me?**

You're not crazy. You're not lazy. You're not just getting old. You're navigating a hormonal hellscape in a neurodivergent brain that was never meant to play by the rules of polite society. Welcome to the party. You're right on time.

New research confirms what AFAB neurodivergent folks have known all along: hormonal transitions like perimenopause and menopause can amplify executive dysfunction, sensory sensitivities, emotional dysregulation, and working memory struggles—especially for those with ADHD and/or autism (Dorani et al., 2021; Kooij et al., 2025; Roberts et al., 2018).

Studies now highlight that perimenopause can actually unmask underlying neurodivergence, which is one reason so many women in particular (and ultimately anyone born with an ovarian system) are diagnosed with ADHD or autism later in life (ADDitude, 2024). This chapter is about making the invisible visible so you can stop doubting yourself and start advocating from a place of clarity.

What You'll Find in Chapter 1:

☑ Detailed **Neuro-Hormonal Decoder Chart**

☑ "You're Not Imagining It" **Dismissal Translation Checklist**

☑ Comprehensive **Neuro-Hormonal Profile Worksheet**

☑ **32 Self-Affirmation Cards** (available in the Online Toolbox ... scan the QR code on page 24 to access your folder of printables.)

Chapter 1 shows you how to make sense of it. The Neuro-Hormonal Decoder helps you pinpoint your symptoms, validate your experiences, and reframe your self-understanding.

⚡ Quickstart Instructions

1 Decode Your Symptoms: Use the Neuro-Hormonal Chaos Decoder Chart to see exactly how your symptoms align and intersect with hormonal and neuro-transmitter changes.

2 Validate Your Experiences: Counteract gaslighting with the "You're Not Imagining It" Checklist.

3 Create Clarity: Fill out your personal Neuro-Hormonal Profile Worksheet.

4 Reinforce Daily: Choose your favorite Affirmation Cards to remind you—you're not alone or broken.

First, a story...

I Thought I Had Early-Onset Dementia ... Turns Out It Was Midlife Hormones + ADHD

There was a stretch of time in my 40s—longer than I care to admit—when I was convinced something was seriously wrong with my brain. I couldn't remember names of people I'd known for years. I'd walk into a room and forget why I was there. Mid-sentence, the word I *just* had on the tip of my tongue would vanish like smoke. And it wouldn't come back. The harder I tried to hold onto thoughts, the more slippery they became.

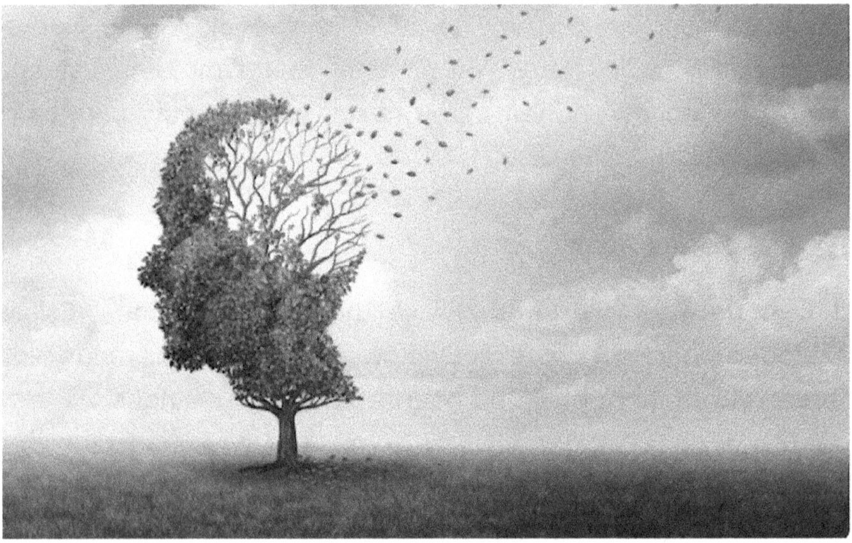

Then came the emotions. I'd cry in the car because I forgot to get tomatoes at the grocery store. Or because the clerk at the post office "scolded" me for filling out a customs form for the package I was mailing incorrectly. Or because I rage-cleaned the entire kitchen after work and not only did no one notice, they immediately made messes everywhere that sent me into tailspins.

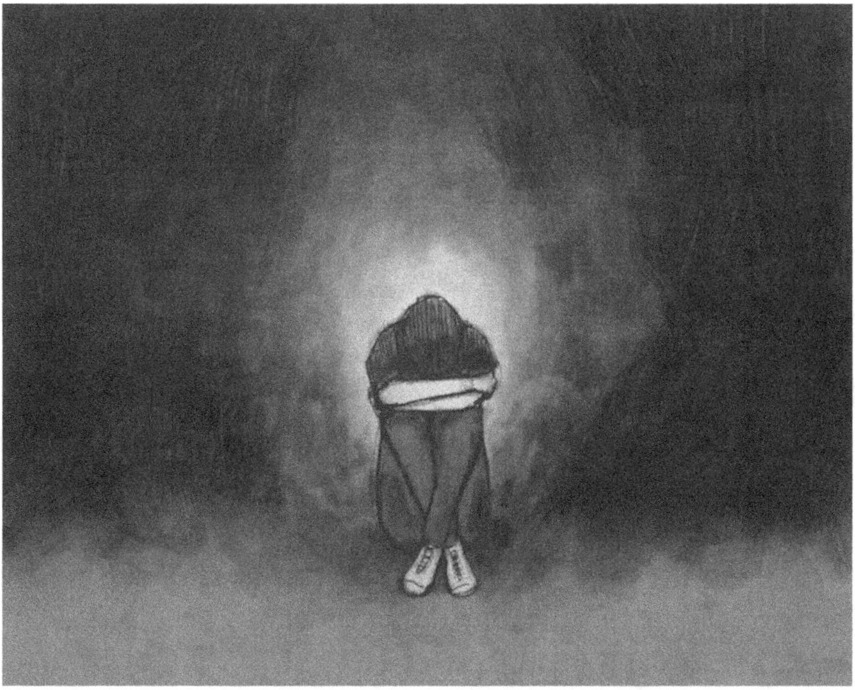

Instead of feeling accomplished, I ended up feeling like a tired old troll yelling at my family for being slobs.

It felt like my mind was short-circuiting. And for a while, I genuinely wondered: *Is this early-onset dementia? Is this what losing yourself feels like? It was legit frightening, and I seriously believed this might be happening to me.*

Turns out, it was a cocktail of midlife hormone chaos and the not-so-fun parts of ADHD and OCD. Estrogen and dopamine were both in short supply, and executive dysfunction was throwing a party I didn't RSVP to. The result? Emotional dysregulation galore.

Unlike you, I didn't have access to a toolkit like this. My doctors and therapists never once considered I might be neurodiver-

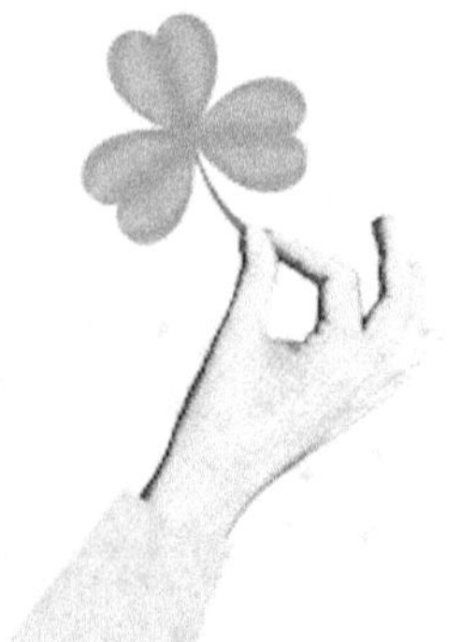

gent, and even though I was given a hormone test in my 40s, it came back normal, and so any thoughts of offering me MHT (menopause hormone therapy), etc. were off the table.

By the time I realized there was a *reason*—a scientific, physiological reason—I was already past menopause and had just gotten my ADHD diagnosis. I had raw-dogged the worst of it. Nevertheless, discovering that all that suffering had reasons felt like someone turned the lights back on. I wasn't broken. I wasn't lazy. I wasn't losing it. I was just midlife-ing with a brain that needed a little more understanding and actual nuanced and targeted treatments. I really could have used a guide like this back then.

✨ *Want more stories like this? Tune into the* ADHD Peri Punks Podcast *and subscribe to ADHD Peri Punks on* SubStack *for solidarity, science, useful tips, and enough laugh-crying to get you through the week. It's free.*

On the following pages, you'll find your ***Neuro-Hormonal Chaos Decoder Symptom Charts***. Now go grab a pencil, and brace yourself for some clarity. You can also find the charts and cards in this book in printable format Online. Just scan the QR code.

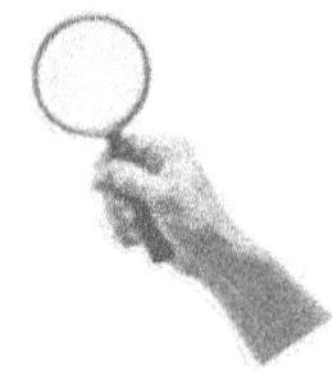

Neuro-Hormonal Chaos Decoder

HIGHLIGHT OR CIRCLE YOUR SYMPTOMS

↓ = DECLINING, DECREASE IN, LOW *↑ = RISING, INCREASE IN, HIGH*

SYMPTOM	HORMONE/ NEURO-TRANSMITTER	WHAT'S GOING ON	WHAT IT FEELS LIKE
INSOMNIA / SLEEP DISTURBANCES	↓ ESTROGEN + PROGESTERONE ↑ CORTISOL	RACING THOUGHTS, HYPERAROUSAL	"3 AM BRAIN REVIEWS EMBARRASSING MOMENTS OR BRILLIANT IDEAS."
EXECUTIVE DYSFUNCTION	↓ ESTROGEN + DOPAMINE	DIFFICULTY STARTING TASKS, STAYING FOCUSED	"WHY DOES REPLYING TO AN EMAIL FEEL LIKE THE ROLLER DERBY?
ELECTRIC SKIN SHOCKS	↓ ESTROGEN ↑ NOREPINEPHRINE	ANXIETY + HYPER-STIMULATION	SUDDEN, BRIEF ZAPS, TINGLING, SENSATIONS UNDER SKIN.
ALLERGY FLARE-UPS	↓ ESTROGEN ↑ HISTAMINE	IMMUNE HYPER-REACTIVITY	WORSENED OR INTENSIFIED ALLERGIES.
DIZZINESS	↓ ESTROGEN + SEROTONIN	INNER-EAR FLUID CHANGES, BLOOD PRESSURE FLUCTUATIONS	FEELING OFF-BALANCE, FREQUENT LIGHTHEADEDNESS.
HEART PALPITATIONS	↓ ESTROGEN ↑ NOREPINEPHRINE	SUDDEN ADRENALINE SURGES	UNEXPECTEDLY RAPID, STRONG HEARTBEAT.
ANXIETY SPIKES	↓ ESTROGEN + GABA ↑ CORTISOL	HYPERAROUSAL	"EVERYTHING FEELS LIKE IT MIGHT GO WRONG AT ONCE. I'M DOOMED."
SUGAR CRAVINGS	↓ ESTROGEN, PROGESTERONE, SEROTONIN, LEPTIN + ENDORPHINS	STRESS EATING; MANAGING CRAVINGS MORE CHALLENGING	"I WILL ABSOLUTELY HAVE MY CAKE AND EAT IT, TOO. WITH A GIANT GLASS OF WINE."
DIGESTIVE ISSUES / BLOATING	↓ ESTROGEN + PROGESTERONE ↑ CORTISOL	GUT-BRAIN AXIS DISRUPTION	"MY STOMACH HAS TURNED INTO A 5-COURSE MEAL BABY, AND IT'S KICKING."

Neuro-Hormonal Chaos Decoder

HIGHLIGHT OR CIRCLE YOUR SYMPTOMS

↓ = DECLINING, DECREASE IN, LOW ↑ = RISING, INCREASE IN, HIGH

SYMPTOM	HORMONE/ NEURO-TRANSMITTER	WHAT'S GOING ON	WHAT IT FEELS LIKE
IRRITABILITY & ANGRY OUTBURSTS	↓ ESTROGEN, PROGESTERONE, + SEROTONIN	LOWER EMOTIONAL REGULATION	QUICK TO FRUSTRATION, EASILY TRIGGERED. "I JUST SCREAMED AT THE CABINET DOOR."
MOOD SWINGS	↓ ESTROGEN, PROGESTERONE, SEROTONIN + DOPAMINE	INTENSE "ILLOGICAL" REACTIONS, SUDDEN, UNCON-TROLLABLE LAUGHTER, CRYING, IRRITABILITY, ETC.	YESTERDAY I WAS FINE. TODAY I'M SOBBING IN THE CAR.
FULL-ON RAGE	↓ ESTROGEN + SEROTONIN	ZERO EMOTIONAL BUFFER, ZERO FILTER	"I DARE YOU TO FUCK WITH ME AND FIND OUT..."
EMOTIONAL FLOODING / TEARS FOR 'NO REASON'	↓ ESTROGEN, PROGESTERONE, + SEROTONIN	OVERWHELMED CIRCUITS, EMOTIONAL CONTROL DISRUPTION	"I CRIED AT A CAR INSURANCE COMMERCIAL."
LOW MOTIVATION/ APATHY	↓ ESTROGEN + DOPAMINE	REWARD CIRCUIT DAMPENING	"I WANT TO CARE. I JUST... DON'T."
SOCIAL EXHAUSTION/ MASKING FATIGUE	↓ ESTROGEN ↑ CORTISOL	PERFORMANCE BURNOUT	"SMALL TALK IS A FULL-BODY WORKOUT."
LOW LIBIDO	↓ ESTROGEN, TESTOSTERONE + DOPAMINE	LACK OF DESIRE	INTIMACY FEELS EXHAUSTING; INTEREST AT AN ALL-TIME LOW. "SEX? NAH, I'M GOOD."
WORD RETRIEVAL ISSUES	↓ ESTROGEN + DOPAMINE	RETRIEVAL GLITCHES	WORDS VANISH MID-CONVO: "THAT THING... WHAT THE HELL IS IT CALLED? THE THING...
MEMORY LAPSES/ LOSING THINGS	↓ ESTROGEN + DOPAMINE	DISRUPTED RECALL	"I HAD MY KEYS, GLASSES, AND COFFEE FIVE SECONDS AGO."

Neuro-Hormonal Chaos Decoder

HIGHLIGHT OR CIRCLE YOUR SYMPTOMS

↓ = DECLINING, DECREASE IN, LOW *↑ = RISING, INCREASE IN, HIGH*

SYMPTOM	HORMONE/ NEURO-TRANSMITTER	WHAT'S GOING ON	WHAT IT FEELS LIKE
BRAIN FOG	↓ ESTROGEN, DOPAMINE + ACETYLCHOLINE	EXECUTIVE DYSFUNCTION	I KNOW I'M FORGETTING SOMETHING IMPORTANT, BUT WTF IS IT?!"
INATTENTIVENESS, DIFFICULTY FOCUSING	↓ DOPAMINE + NOREPINEPHRINE	DISTRACTIBILITY, MENTAL DRFIT	"I READ THIS PARAGRAPH 7 TIMES. STILL NO IDEA WHAT IT SAYS."
IMPULSIVITY (SHOPPING, BINGE-EATING, ETC.)	↓ DOPAMINE + SEROTONIN	POOR IMPULSE CONTROL, ENGAGING IN RISKY BEHAVIOR OR ACTING IN ANGER WITHOUT CONSIDERING THE IMPACT.	CRUISES AMAZON AT 3AM. SEES BULK BOX OF 12 BAGS OF CHIPS. ADDS TO CART. PAYS EXTRA FOR 3 HOUR SHIPPING. CHIPS ARRIVE. EATS 3 BAGS FOR BREAKFAST.
COMPULSIVE BEHAVIOR	↓ DOPAMINE + SEROTONIN ↑ CORTISOL	REPEATED ACTIONS TO QUELL ANXIETY, E.G. EXCESSIVE EXERCISING/ENDORPHIN ADDICTION	WHEN YOU LITERALLY RUN FOR YOUR LIFE. THEM: "HOW DO YOU STAY SO THIN?" ME: "ANXIETY."
INTERNAL HYPER-ACTIVITY	↓ ESTROGEN + DOPAMINE	MENTAL RESTLESSNESS, SELF-PRESSURE, INTERRUPTS OTHERS	"I'M SITTING STILL BUT MY BRAIN IS AT A RAVE."
AUDITORY SENSITIVITY	↓ ESTROGEN + GABA	AUDITORY FILTERING DIFFICULTY	"THAT HUMMING FLUORESCENT LIGHT IS MY PERSONAL HELL."
AUDITORY INFO PROCESSING DELAYS	↓ GABA, DOPAMINE ↓ SEROTONIN, OR JUST A GENERAL IMBALANCE ↓ OR ↑ GLUTAMATE	DELAYED RESPONSE TO SENSORY STIMULI; YOUR HEARING IS FINE BUT IT SEEMS LIKE YOU'RE NOT LISTENING	"I'M NOT BEING RUDE AND NO, I'M NOT DEAF. MY BRAIN JUST NEEDS MORE TIME TO PROCESS WHAT YOU'RE SAYING."
ITCHY EARS	↓ ESTROGEN + COLLAGEN ↓ PROGESTERONE IN FLUX	REDUCED NATURAL OIL PRODUCTION	AN ANNOYING ITCH THAT'S IMPOSSIBLE TO SCRATCH.
TINNITUS	↓ ESTROGEN + SEROTONIN	AUDITORY NERVE SENSITIVITY INCREASED	PERSISTENT RINGING, BUZZING, WHOOSHING IN EARS.

Neuro-Hormonal Chaos Decoder

HIGHLIGHT OR CIRCLE YOUR SYMPTOMS

↓ = DECLINING, DECREASE IN, LOW ↑ = RISING, INCREASE IN, HIGH

SYMPTOM	HORMONE/ NEURO-TRANSMITTER	WHAT'S GOING ON	WHAT IT FEELS LIKE
NEED FOR ROUTINE / TRANSITIONS FEEL HARD	↓ DOPAMINE + SEROTONIN	CHANGE DYSREGULATION	SOMEONE MOVED MY MUG AND MY THERAPIST CHANGED MY APPT. TIME THIS WEEK. I AM NOT OK.
REPETITIVE STIMMING BEHAVIORS	↓ ESTROGEN, SEROTONIN + GABA	STRONG URGE TO USE MOVEMENTS AS A REGULATION TOOL FOR MANAGING EMOTIONS AND SENSORY INPUT	TAPPING, FIDGETING, NAIL BITING, CHEWING ON PENS, JEWELRY, ETC. SUCKING/BITING CHEEKS, LIPS, REPETITIVE MOUTH MOVEMENTS OR SOUNDS
SENSORY OVERLOAD / SENSITIVITY	↓ ESTROGEN, GABA + SEROTONIN	HEIGHTENED SENSRY GATING MALFUNCTION	CLOTHING IS PAINFUL, SOUNDS ARE UNBEARBALE, LIGHTS ARE TOO BRIGHT. "THE TAG ON MY SHIRT IS PURE EVIL."
REJECTION SENSITIVITY DYSPHORIA (RSD)	↓ DOPAMINE + NOREPINEPHRINE ↑ CORTISOL	EMOTIONAL PAIN FROM PERCEIVED REJECTION	"WHY AREN'T THEY TEXTING ME RIGHT BACK? DID I DO SOMETHING WRONG? WHAT DID I DO? I'M A SHIT PERSON."
TEMPERATURE DYSREGULATION (HOT FLASHES & NIGHT SWEATS)	↓ ESTROGEN ↗ SEROTONIN FLUCTUATIONS ↑ NOREPINEPHRINE	HYPOTHALAMUS OVERREACTS, TEMPERATURE REGULATION CHAOS	SUDDEN HEAT WAVES, SWEATING EPISODES FOLLOWED BY IMMEDIATE CHILLS. "HEY, I'M A VOLCANO...WAIT, NOW I'M AN ICEBERG!"
GENITAL DRYNESS (PAINFUL SEX IF SEXUALLY ACTIVE)	↓ ESTROGEN + TESTOSTERONE	REDUCED MOISTURE AND LESS ELASTICITY; SHAME AND/OR DYSPHORIA TRIGGERING POSSIBLE	INTIMACY UNCOMFORT-ABLE OR PAINFUL. MAY DISRUPT RELATIONSHIP. "MY POOL MEMBERSHIP LAPSED AND RELOCATED ME TO THE DESERT WITHOUT TELLING ME."
GLUTEAL TENDINOPATHY, HIP PAIN, SCIATICA	↓ ESTROGEN + COLLAGEN AS A RESULT	SOFT TISSUE VULNERABILITY, CONNECTIVE TISSUE STIFF-NESS, TENDON DEGENERATION, IMFLAMMATION	PERSISTENT OUTER HIP PAIN, DIFFICULTY SITTING OR LYING ON SIDE, RADIATING NERVE PAIN DOWN LEG, TROUBLE SITTING/ DRIVING, ETC.

Neuro-Hormonal Chaos Decoder

HIGHLIGHT OR CIRCLE YOUR SYMPTOMS

↓ = DECLINING, DECREASE IN, LOW ↑ = RISING, INCREASE IN, HIGH

SYMPTOM	HORMONE/ NEURO-TRANSMITTER	WHAT'S GOING ON	WHAT IT FEELS LIKE
JOINT PAIN, BODY ACHES, FROZEN SHOULDER	↓ ESTROGEN + COLLAGEN AS A RESULT	SENSORY AMPLIFICATION, INCREASED INFLAMMATION	"I DID NOTHING AND MY KNEES ARE LITERALLY YELLING AT ME."
HAIR LOSS / THINNING	↓ ESTROGEN, POSSIBLE TESTO-STERONE + POTENTIALLY HYPOACTIVE THYROXINE (T4) & TRIIODOTHYRONINE (T3) AKA THYROID HORMONES	REDUCED HAIR FOLLICLE STRENGTH, VISIBLE AGING, IDENTITY SHIFT	SIGNIFICANT SHEDDING, LESS VOLUME. "WHO CLOGGED THE SHOWER DRAIN? WELL SHIT... I DID."
BRITTLE NAILS	↓ ESTROGEN + TESTOSTERONE	REDUCED COLLAGEN & KERATIN STRENGTH	NAILS THAT BREAK OR PEEL EASILY
INCREASED BELLY FAT	↓ ESTROGEN	BELLY FAT ACCUMULATES DESPITE NO MAJOR CHANGES IN DIET & EXERCISE	"HUH. THIS MUFFIN I ATE FOR BREAKFAST MULTIPLIED AND TRANSFERRED ITSELF TO MY LOWER ABDOMEN."
CHEST & NIPPLE PAIN / TENDER-NESS, CHANGES IN CHEST SHAPE OR VOLUME	↓ ESTROGEN + PROGESTERONE ↑ PROLACTIN SURGE POSSIBLE	DISCOMFORT FROM EVEN MILD CLOTHING FRIC-TION; INTRUSIVE FOCUS ON BODILY CHANGES; ANXIET ABOUT APPEARANCE	"MY BODY HAS DECIDED TO REBRAND WITHOUT MY CONSENT. GRAVITY IS NOT MY FRIEND."
IRREGULAR PERIODS SHORTER, LIGHTER, LESS FREQUENT OR HEAVIER, LONGER, MORE FREQUENT (TO CONFUSE YOU) OR **NO PERIOD FOR 1+ YEAR**	↓ ESTROGEN + PROGESTERONE	EXACERBATED SYMPTOMS, IMPACT ON DAILY LIFE IS SIGNIFICANT, DELAYED NEURODEVELOP-MENTAL DIAGNOSES DUE TO OVERLAPPING SYMPTOMS	"I AM IN HELL. MY EXISTING SENSITIVITIES AND COPING MECHANISMS ARE STRETCHED TO THEIR LIMITS. EVERYONE THINKS I'M BATSHIT CRAZY, AND NO ONE IS LISTENING TO ME."

Neuro-Hormonal Chaos Decoder

HIGHLIGHT OR CIRCLE YOUR SYMPTOMS

↓ = DECLINING, DECREASE IN, LOW   *↑ = RISING, INCREASE IN, HIGH*

SYMPTOM	PANIC ATTACKS / SEVERE ANXIETY	SUICIDAL IDEATION AND/OR SELF-HARM
HORMONE/ NEURO-TRANSMITTER	↕ ESTROGEN, PROGESTERONE + SEROTONIN FLUCTUATIONS & DYSREGULATED DOPAMINE ↑ NOREPINEPHRINE SURGE	↓ ESTROGEN, PROGESTERONE + DOPAMINE ↕ SEROTONIN DYSREGULATION ↑ CORTISOL SPIKES
WHAT'S GOING ON	TYPICAL STRESSORS SUDDENLY FEEL URGENT. A GROCERY STORE AISLE FEELS LIKE A WAR ZONE; THE SOUND OF A CHECKOUT BEEP CAN TIP YOU INTO FULL-ON FIGHT-OR-FLIGHT. FOR ND BRAINS USED TO RACING THOUGHTS, THIS PANIC IS NEXT-LEVEL. YOUR CHEST FEELS TIGHT, YOUR ARMS FEEL NUMB AND TINGLY. YOUR HEART RATE SPIKES. YOU HYPERVENTILATE. YOU LEGIT THINK YOU'RE DYING.	INTENSIFIED HOPELESSNESS, EMOTIONAL DYSREGULATION, DIFFICULTY ACCESSING LOGICAL PERSPECTIVE; YOU MAY MISINTERPRET THESE SHIFTS AS PERMANENT OR PERSONAL FAILINGS; DARK, INTRUSIVE THOUGHTS THAT FEEL LIKE THEY DON'T BELONG TO YOU. FOR MANY NEURODIVERGENT BRAINS ALREADY PRIMED FOR RUMINATION, REJECTION SENSITIVITY, AND EMOTIONAL WHIPLASH, THE HORMONAL STORM OF PERIMEMOPAUSE POURS GASOLINE ON A FIRE YOU DIDN'T START.
WHAT IT FEELS LIKE	RECURRING SENSE OF DOOM & CHEST TIGHTNESS; YOUR OWN NERVOUS SYSTEM HAS STAGED A COUP. ONE MINUTE YOU'RE CHOOSING A BAG OF APPLES, THE NEXT, YOU'RE CLUTCHING YOUR CHEST, CONVINCED YOU'RE HAVING A HEART ATTACK. CUE THE SPIRAL: "WHAT IF I DIE RIGHT HERE? WHAT IF I NEVER SEE MY KIDS/PARTNER/FAMILY AGAIN?" THE TERROR IS SO REAL, YOU COULD CRY, SCREAM, OR BOTH. YOU ARE PARALYZED BY FEAR & FEEL HELPLESS.	A RELENTLESS MENTAL LOOP IN THE NEGATIVE SPACE: "WHAT IF I CAN'T KEEP GOING? WHAT IF EVERYONE WOULD BE BETTER OFF WITHOUT ME?" *** THIS IS SERIOUS. EVEN IF YOU'VE NEVER FELT SUICIDAL BEFORE, THE SUDDENNESS & INTENSITY OF THESE THOUGHTS CAN BE TERRIFYING. IF YOU'RE HAVING THOUGHTS OF ENDING YOUR LIFE OR HARMING YOURSELF, YOU'RE NOT BROKEN. YOU'RE NOT ALONE. YOU ARE EXPERIENCING BIOCHEMICAL CHANGES THAT AFFECT MOOD & COGNITION. YOU DESERVE IMMEDIATE SUPPORT.

If you or someone you know is suicidal, call or text the suicide hotline in your country. If someone is in IMMEDIATE danger, please call your local emergency number (e.g. 911 in the US).

US & Canada: Emergency: 911; Suicide Hotline: 988

UK & Ireland: Emergency: 999; Suicide Hotline: 116 123

Australia: Emergency: 000; Suicide Hotline: 13 11 14

Bahamas: Emergency 911; Suicide Hotline (2) 322-2763

Barbados: Emergency 911: Suicide Hotline: (246) 4299999

Jamaica: Emergency police: 119; Medical Emergency: 110; Suicide Hotline: (888) 639-5433

South Africa: Emergency police: 10111; Medical Emergency: 10177; Suicide Hotline: 0800 567 567

New Zealand: Emergency: 111; Suicide Hotline: 0800 543 354

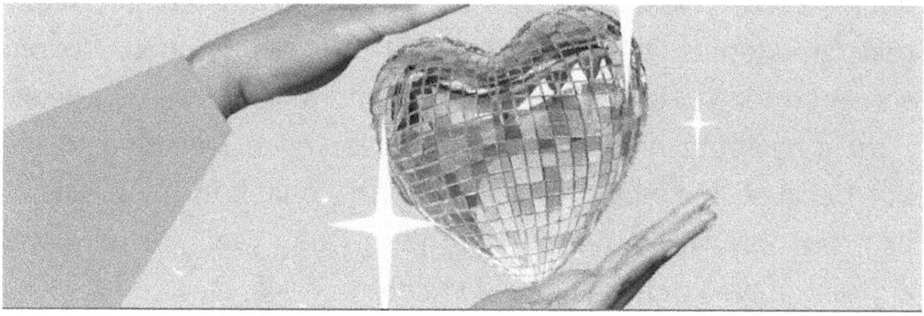

YOU ARE NOT CRAZY. AND YOU ARE NOT ALONE.

* * *

I wish someone had told me years ago that suicidal thoughts in perimenopause are not a moral failing—they're a neurological and hormonal crisis. The data are sobering: suicide rates for women peak in midlife from hormonal shifts alone, and the risk can be greater for neurodivergent women because ADHD, autism, and OCD already carry higher baseline rates of self-harm and suicidal ideation, especially if left undiagnosed and untreated (Chapman et al., 2025; Hendriks et al., 2025).

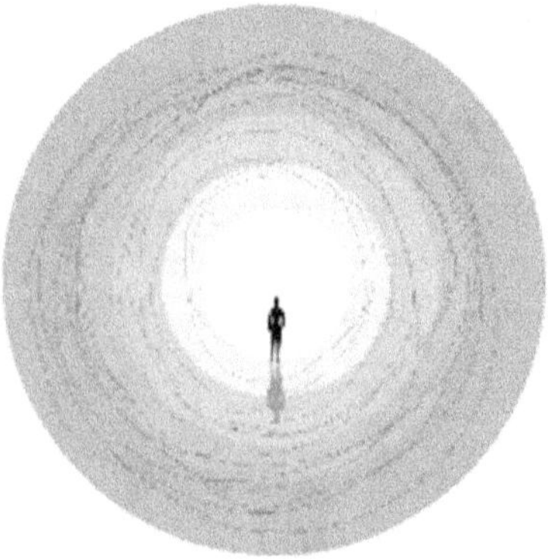

For most of my 30s and 40s, I was prescribed antidepressants, antipsychotics, and sedatives for what was labeled treatment-resistant depression. No one asked about hormones. No one screened for ADHD or OCD. And yet, there were intervals where I thought about ending my life—not because I wanted to die, but because the idea of relief from the chaos in my brain felt like the only way out. The only thing that kept me here was knowing it would devastate my children.

Two years+ into proper ADHD and OCD treatment, combined with hormone replacement therapy for estrogen decline, I feel like my-self again. This isn't a push for HRT; it's a call to help you find what works best for you. If you're in that dark place, please know this: you are not crazy, not broken, and not beyond help. It's not you—it's your brain chemistry. And it can change.

References:

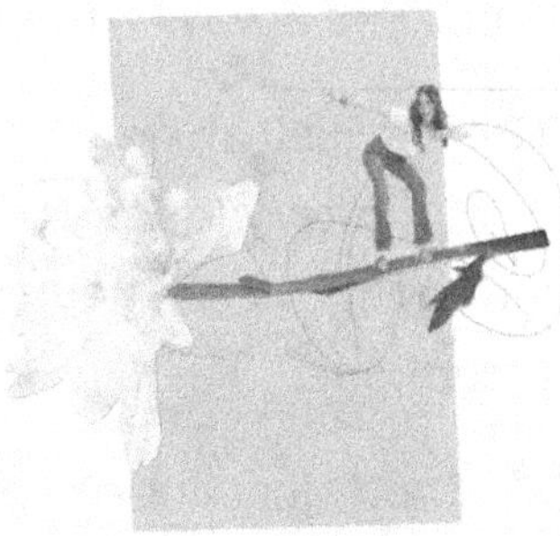

Chapman, S. et al. (2025). Examining the link between ADHD symptoms and menopausal experiences. *Journal of Attention Disorders.*

Hendriks, O. et al. (2025). The mental health challenges, especially suicidality, experienced by women during perimenopause and menopause: A qualitative study. *Women's health (London, England), 21,* 17455057251338941.

🚫 You're Not Imagining It: Symptom & Gaslight Checklist Common Dismissals & Their Reality

"Transform every dismissal into validation."

❌ "It's just stress." → It's not "just" stress. It's hormonal + neurological.

❌ "You're too young for menopause." → Perimenopause symptoms can begin by age 35.

❌ "Everyone forgets things." → Not like this. This cognitive disruption is deeper and hormonal.

❌ "You just need yoga." → Yes, yoga is awesome for some people. But. Yoga won't regulate hormones or dopamine. Hormonal dysregulation isn't fixed by mindfulness alone.

❌ "You're too sensitive." → Sensory processing changes are real. Perimenopause neurologically amplifies everything.

❌ "Your labs are normal." → Functionality (or lack thereof) + symptoms always trumps numerical results.

❌ "It's just anxiety." → This isn't "just" "worry." It's multi-system hormonal and neurotransmitter disruptions.

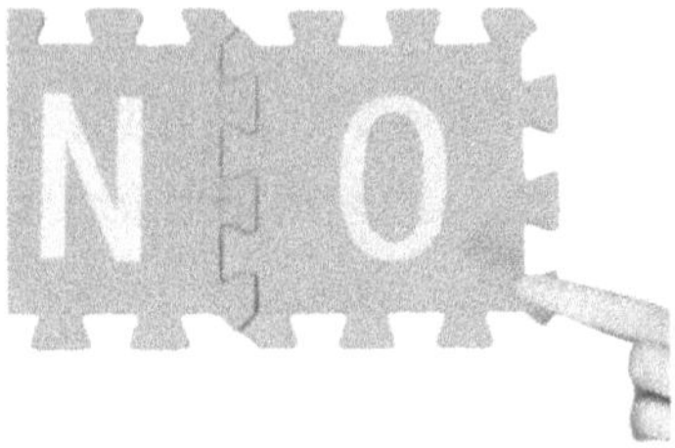

❌ "You just need better time management." → No planner fixes executive dysfunction.

❌ "You should lose weight." → Irrelevant. Also: stop.

❌ "You're overreacting." → Nope.

❌ "You're just getting older." → Common does not mean acceptable.

❌ "But you're successful, so it can't be that bad." → Success can mask suffering.

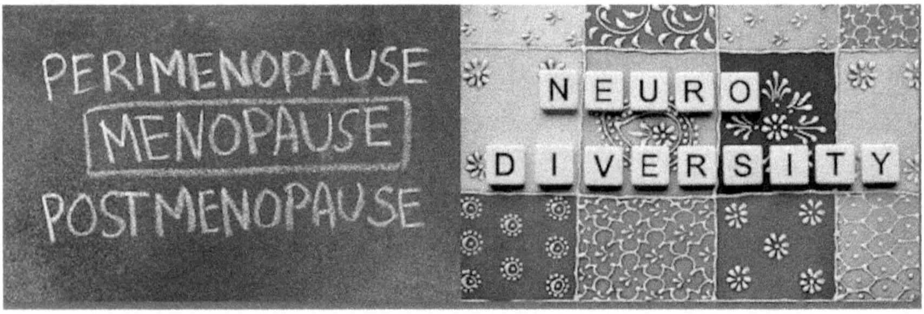

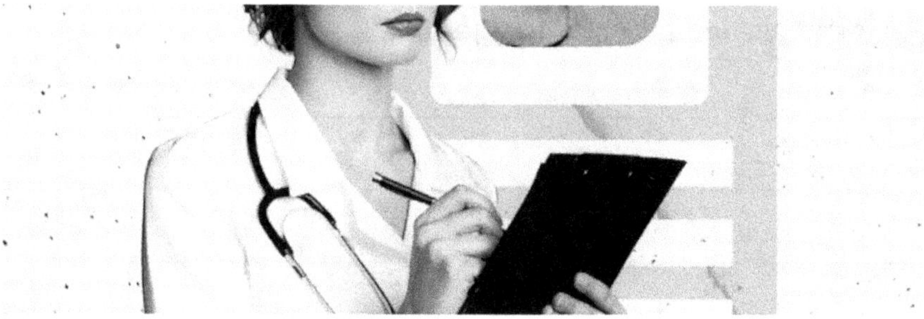

My Neuro-Hormonal Profile Worksheet

Who TF Am I Right Now?

Age: ________

Diagnosis/Suspected: ADHD / Autistic / Both / Other / Unsure

Top 5 Symptoms:

1.

2.

3.

4.

5.

* * *

Patterns Noticed (cycle, triggers):

____

____

____

____

____

What Helps (even a little):

1. ____

2. ____

3. ____

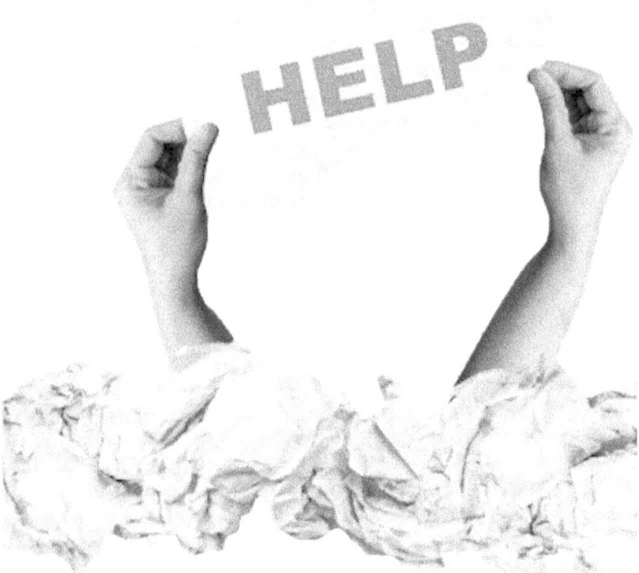

. . .

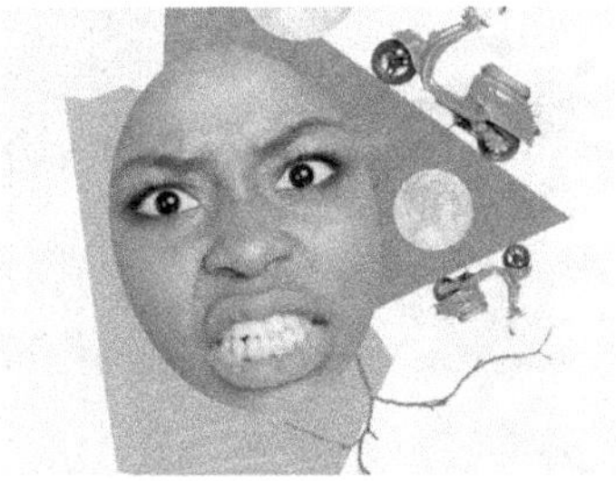

What Makes Everything Worse:

1. ______________________________

2. ______________________________

3. ______________________________

Three Things My Medical Provider Must Hear:

1. ____

2. ____

3. ____

Bring this. Hand it over. Walk out taller.

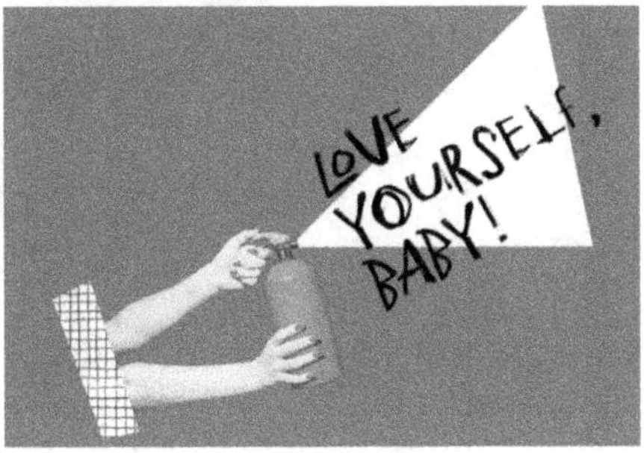

Next up: **32 affirmations** to remind you that you aren't disordered. The system is. Print and cut these if you're feeling crafty. Use a thicker cardstock to get a deck effect!

QR code on the following page! Yes, again.

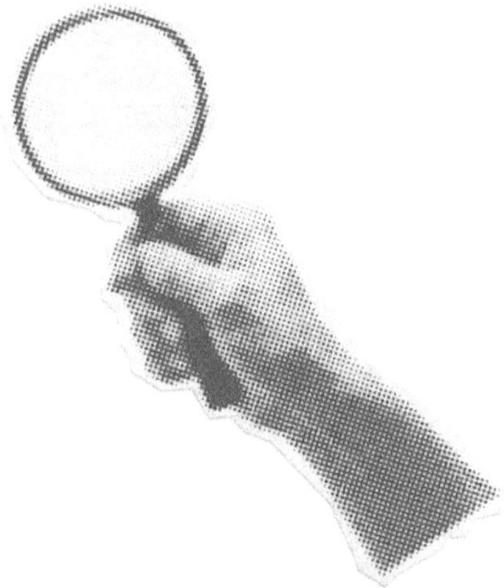

Don't forget to remember! All cards, charts, scripts, etc. in this book are available to download and/or print in your own Online toolbox.

1. My brain isn't broken. My estrogen is.

2. I'm not crazy. I'm out of fucking neurotransmitters

3. This is a hormonal hostage situation.

4. My burnout is not a personality flaw.

1 You're not losing it. You're navigating a biologically brutal system without a map. This toolkit is your map.

2 Low dopamine. Low serotonin. Low estrogen. High expectations. You're allowed to fall apart.

3 You're doing your best while your body throws flaming hormonal knives. You're still here. That's badass.

4 You're not lazy, weak, or broken. You've been doing life on Hard Mode without instructions.

5 I didn't forget. My memory is on strike.

6 I am not "too much." Others are underprepared.

7 My body is loud because it needs care.

8 I have nothing to prove today.

5 Memory loss isn't a moral failure. It's a biological side effect. And yes, write it down 87 times.

6 You've just outgrown everyone's tiny boxes and fragile egos. Stay big.

7 Pain, fatigue, rage — all love notes saying, "Pay attention to me."

8 Being alive is already a full-time job. You can rest now.

9 Panic isn't weakness. It's a red flag signaling for help.

10 Crying isn't failure. It's release.

11 My worth isn't tied to my productivity.

12 This fog doesn't erase who I am.

9 Your nervous system needs calm, not shame. Breathe like you deserve it.

10 You're not dramatic — you're defrosting years of bottled-up cortisol.

11 Your value doesn't drop when your to-do list stays full. Sometimes you just gotta kick that list to the curb!

12 You're still brilliant, even if your brain feels like scrambled eggs today. Or a fried one...this is your brain on years of undiagnosed neurodivergence + peri/menopause.

13 I deserve real answers, not bullshit platitudes.

14 I don't have to mask here.

15 My feelings are data, not drama.

16 I don't owe anyone my silence.

13 If one more doctor says "just relax," you have my permission to hiss.

14 You're safe. Take off the people-pleasing costume and breathe.

15 If it feels big to you, it IS big. Trust yourself, beautiful human.

16 Take up space. Use your outside voice. You're allowed.

17 I trust my lived experience.

18 Sensory overload is not "too sensitive."

19 My body is not the enemy.

20 Anger is a boundary, not a flaw.

17 If your gut and Google agree — you're probably right.

18 You're not delicate — you're operating without filters in a loud world.

19 You're tired, not traitorous. Feed yourself, move, love yourself anyway.

20 Rage is your nervous system saying, "Something's not right here."

21 I am allowed to be inconvenient.

22 Sleep is not laziness.

23 I can't outwork my hormones — and that's okay.

24 I am worthy of care right now.

21 You don't exist to make other people comfortable.

22 Recovery is rebellious in a world that worships hustle.

23 You don't need to earn rest. You already deserve it. Rest is resistance, a neurobiological imperative you don't have to earn.

24 Not when you're "better." Not when you "fix" it. Now.

25 I deserve community, not isolation.

26 Self-care is my quiet rebellion.

27 This pain doesn't define me.

28 Even when I feel invisible, I matter.

25 Humans are pack animals. You're not meant to do this alone.

26 Light a candle. Take a nap. Delete the email. No apologies. Self care is community care, bitches.

27 It's a chapter, not the whole damn book.

28 Just because they don't see you doesn't mean you disappeared.

29 I don't have to explain myself to everyone.

30 Healing is punk as hell.

31 Stop screaming into pillows.

32 Your rage is valid and needs to be uncaged.

29 "No" is a complete sentence. Use it.

30 Getting back up every day IS the revolution.

31 You deserve to be heard, not muted.

32 Go outside, raise your face up to the sky, fists pumped, and release your rage like a first-time mom in labor with triplets and no epidural.

🩶 Wrap-Up / Next Steps

You just made the invisible visible—and that's power. Print your profile. Say the damn affirmations. Stick them everywhere. You're not imagining this. You're decoding it, and you've taken the first step toward radical clarity.

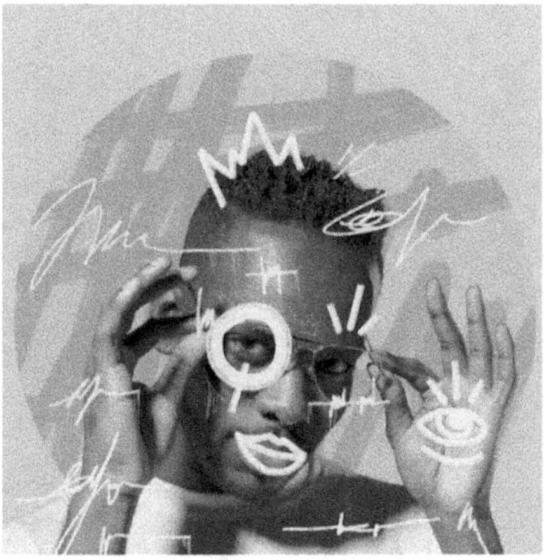

Next Up: Self-Advocacy Simplified

Because we're not crying in doctors' offices anymore—we're coming in armed with data. We've logged our symptoms, and we know we have options. You've clarified your experience—now you have language and evidence. This visibility is powerful.

Now, transform clarity into actionable strategies with your providers.

This book was conceptualized, designed and written by someone not unlike you: overstimulated, underdiagnosed, and absolutely DONE with medical gaslighting. Welcome to your clarity era.

Chapter 2

Self-Advocacy Simplified

Theme: Empowerment

Goal: Help you walk into medical, workplace, or family conversations armed with language, tools, and confidence—so you can get the care and respect you deserve.

* * *

We're not crying in doctors' offices anymore.
We're walking in with data, research, and a perfectly polite "try me."

The System Is Still Behind, So Here's How We Stay Ahead

Despite growing awareness, medical care for midlife cis women —especially those who are neurodivergent—is still riddled with gaps. For gender-expansive and nonbinary folks, Black, Brown, Indigenous? Indeed, gender-diverse populations have been neglected, and People of the Global Majority are ironically exponentially underfunded and understudied. Studies show that most providers underestimate the cognitive and emotional impact of hormonal changes, and few are trained to recognize how neurodivergence interacts with perimenopause (Kooij et al., 2025; Luine, 2014; Russell et al., 2019).

This chapter equips you with the tools and language to bridge that gap: to demand the care you deserve, to know when to seek second opinions, and to ensure your symptoms aren't dismissed because your labs are "normal."

What You'll Find in Chapter 2:

☑ **Power Principles Guide**

☑ **Symptom Snapshot Sheet**

☑ **Provider Script**

☑ **Appointment Prep Checklist**

☑ **Non-HRT Supplements & Nutrition Guide**

☑ **Movement & Mobility Modifications Guide**

Welcome & Why This Matters

Have you ever rage-cried in your car after a healthcare appointment? Or walked out feeling unheard, unseen, and/or quietly ashamed for even asking for help?

No more.

You're not here to beg for scraps of care anymore — you're here to collaborate. And you're walking in with evidence and a toolkit full of fire.

You are the expert on your own body. When you advocate for yourself, you aren't just getting better care — you're also setting a standard for how you deserve to be treated everywhere.

Chapter 2 teaches you how to:

✔ Reclaim the power dynamic

✔ Speak the right language to get what you need

✔ Document your experience so they can't ignore it

✔ Hold boundaries and (if needed) walk away

⚡ **Quickstart Instructions**

1 Read the Self-Advocacy Power Principles - reset your mindset for medical appointments. Remind yourself why you have the right to be heard, believed, and supported — without apology.

2 Fill Out Your Symptom Snapshot Sheet - get your top concerns crystal clear. Print and complete this before any appointment to clearly capture what you're experiencing and what you want.

3 Review and Practice the Provider Script - walk in with strong language. Use the fill-in-the-blank script to say what you need confidently, even if your hands are shaking.

4 Highlight Your Priorities with the Appointment Prep Checklist - no detail missed. Print the checklist and mark the 1-2 main goals for your visit so you can stay focused when the nerves kick in.

5 Review the non-HRT supplements & nutrition guide - build your baseline health now. Familiarize Yourself with Evidence-Based Options. Look over the notes on MHT, GAHT, non-HRT supplements, lifestyle strategies, and nutrition/movement tips — so you can ask informed questions and make decisions that feel right for you.

6 Plan Your Exit Strategy (if needed). If you're dismissed or minimized? You already know: that's your cue to find a new provider who *deserves* you.

7 Remind yourself daily: You're not asking for a favor. You're asking for the care you deserve.

First, a story...

The Day Christina Refused to Be Dismissed

I met Christina when I was 17 my first semester at college, and we were thick as thieves almost immediately. She was wild, fun, so kind, and the vibrant soul I needed in my life at that time. We don't see each other often, but we are friends to this day, and she's still got that wild and crazy spirit.

But she almost lost it. Christina had always been deeply in tune with her body. So when a sore throat lingered for weeks and exhaustion wrapped itself around her like wet cement at 37, she knew something wasn't right. Her doctor brushed it off—probably just a virus. Weeks passed. She went back, insisted on tests, and was dismissed again.

By the time she sought a second opinion, she was frantic. Same answer: "We can't find anything wrong." That's when her voice broke into something fierce. In the exam room, she shouted through tears, "Then why do I feel so awful?" Still, no answers.

It took a third doctor, at a completely different clinic, to listen without rushing, to run the right in-depth tests. The result? A rare form of lung cancer, unrelated to smoking. For the next year, Christina endured radiation, chemotherapy, and the terrifying uncertainty of a disease that had nearly been ignored into catastrophe.

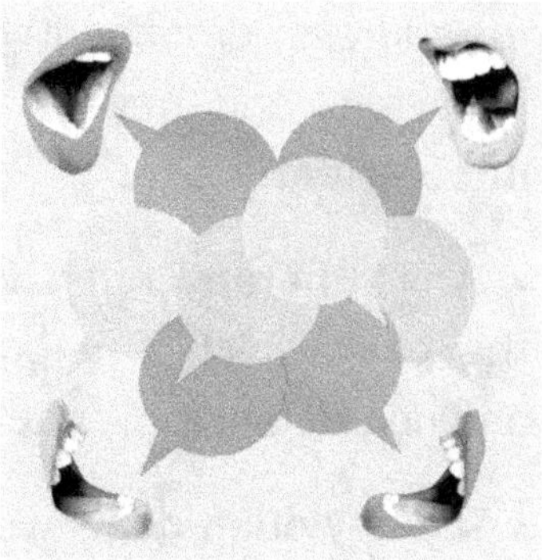

She survived. Today, at 56, she's cancer-free and thriving. But her story is a sharp reminder: self-advocacy can save your life. If you don't feel well, there's always a reason. Keep speaking up until someone listens. You are the expert on your body—and your voice is your most powerful tool.

Building Your Neuroaffirming Healthcare Dream Team

Finding one affirming provider can feel like a victory, but **true support often requires a network.** Menopause and neurodivergence both impact many parts of life—physical, mental, emotional, and social. A single doctor, no matter how skilled, may lack the time or expertise to address everything you bring to the table. Building a team that understands your neurotype(s), respects your lived experience, and adapts to your needs is an act of self-respect. Your general practitioner may oversee broad health issues, but a hormone specialist can help with management and symptom relief. Moreover, **therapists familiar with both neurodivergence and midlife transitions can provide a space to process changes, address mood shifts, and teach emotional regulation.**

Neuroaffirming Therapy and Coaching

Executive Function Coaching as a Powerful Add-on

• **Neuroaffirming therapy** can offer a wide array of approaches to address emotional regulation, self-compassion, masking behaviors, and trauma — making **both meds and coaching more effective.**

• While **therapy** often focuses on unraveling and **processing the past**, which is important for healing and self-compassion and understanding, **coaching** is more **goal-oriented**.

• Therapy often deals with **emotional regulation, insight, and trauma**; coaching focuses on **application** — how to actually get shit done.

• **Executive function** is hands-down one of the more significant challenges for ADHDers and Autistic folks. Even if you're neurodivergent and have been holding it together well enough, the **estrogen fluctuation** that takes dopamine with it during perimenopause can easily rip the mask off and make all the things you used to manage to do exponentially harder. Coaching doesn't treat medically, but rather helps **build practical systems** (planning, time management, follow-through) and **boosts self-efficacy**. A ND-affirming coach may offer practical tools for executive dysfunction or help you unmask safely in your daily routines.

Menopause coaches and therapists exist, too! So do **gender-affirming menopause care providers and consultants.**

Coaches who understand executive (dys)function, peri and menopause and/or genderqueer menopause via their own **lived experience** can translate one or more of these into **tactical strategies** for scheduling, structuring, and building systems that align with neurodivergent brains.

Advantage: You move from "understanding the why" to "operationalizing the how."

Vetting providers takes effort, but it pays off. Early appointments are much like interviews—you are hiring them to care for you. Start by looking for signs of neuroaffirming practice.

- Does this provider listen without interrupting?
- Do they explain terms in plain language and invite your input?
- Are they open to adapting their approach if something does not work for you?

Red flags include dismissiveness, rigid adherence to protocols that ignore your communication needs, or an unwillingness to acknowledge the neurodiversity paradigm and neurodivergence as valid. Prepare a set of questions for new providers:

"How familiar are you with neurodivergent adults?"

"Have you treated patients in menopause who also have ADHD and/or autism (+ other co-morbid conditions)?"

"Are you comfortable adjusting sensory environments or pacing conversations for processing time?"

Watch how they respond. Defensive answers or visible discomfort are clues this may not be the right fit.

Consider who you trust with your stories—sometimes it's a nurse practitioner who listens carefully, a social worker who connects you with resources, or a community health worker who shares your background. **This network is not just about credentials; it's about working with people who see you as a whole person.** If a provider's website mentions trauma-informed care, neurodiversity-affirming practice, or intersectional awareness, these are good signs. Still, nothing replaces your own assessment—trust your instincts if something feels off.

Support networks play a critical role in advocacy. Bringing someone with you—a partner, friend, or advocate—can make appointments safer and less overwhelming. A support buddy serves as another set of ears, helps clarify information, and can take notes when stress makes details hard to remember. **Sometimes their presence alone shifts the power dynamic, signaling to providers that you have backup and will not be brushed aside.** If words escape you or anxiety spikes, your ally can prompt gently: "Was there something else you wanted to discuss?" This collaboration is not overstepping; it is a form of mutual care many people rely on.

Your healthcare dream team will likely evolve as needs change. You may outgrow certain relationships or require different expertise over time. That's natural and healthy. The most important lesson is that you are allowed to expect respect and competence from everyone involved in your care.

Similarly, you are entitled to assert your identity and expect respect in that regard as well. **When misgendered or addressed by the wrong name, calmly but firmly correct the staff**:

"My pronouns are they/them—please use them."

While it can feel vulnerable to do this repeatedly, it sets boundaries that should be honored. **If your symptoms are minimized, state plainly:**

"I need you to take this seriously because it's affecting my health and daily life."

These direct requests might feel bold or uncomfortable, but with time, asserting your needs becomes easier. Many need to take this step for fair treatment.

Discrimination and bias should not be tolerated in silence. If you feel dismissed because of your identity, voice it directly:

"I feel I'm not being heard because of my identity. Who can I speak to about this?"

If you need to file a complaint—about discrimination, unprofessional behavior, or unsafe care—contact the clinic's patient advocate or ombudsman. Keep notes about what happened: dates, names, descriptions. (Have a trusted ally help you compile this.) You can also reach out to professional licensing boards or advocacy organizations for further support. These steps may feel daunting but are sometimes necessary for your protection and the improvement of care for others.

Just remember: Even the best plans sometimes fall apart. If a provider proves unhelpful—minimizing your symptoms, refusing accommodations, or failing to respect your identity—be prepared to move on. You do not owe loyalty to someone who treats you poorly. Signs it is time to switch include repeated dismissal ("It's probably just stress"), lack of improvement despite clear communication, or feeling worse after every visit.

When leaving a provider, request a copy of your records in writing; this is your legal right and will ease transition to new care. Ask for referrals if needed—"Can you recommend someone experienced with neurodivergent adults?" If the situation is urgent or unsafe, seek out emergency helplines or crisis support immediately.

Building a supportive network takes work but provides real benefits: better communication, more tailored treatment, reduced anxiety, and greater safety in medical spaces. You are not alone in needing this kind of holistic support—many find strength in teams rather than solo efforts.

Self-Advocacy Power Principles

These are your ground rules going in:

1 ❏ You're allowed to ask questions. → Informed ≠ difficult.

2 ❏ You don't have to "prove" your pain. → You're not auditioning for care. Function matters more than tests.

3 ❏ Saying "I don't know" is power, not weakness. → Admitting uncertainty helps your provider help you.

4 ❏ Normal labs ≠ normal life. → Function is always more important than numbers. ALWAYS. Also, WTF ? Define *normal*.

5 ❏ "No" is a redirection, not the end. → "No" just means: next doctor. Second (or third) opinions are valid & might be needed.

Symptom Snapshot Sheet

Name/pronouns: ______________________________

Date: ______________________________

1. Top 3 Symptoms

1)

2)

3)

* * *

2. Symptom Frequency & Intensity

1) ____________________ **Daily / Weekly / Monthly**

Severity (0–10):

2) ____________________ **Daily / Weekly / Monthly**

Severity (0–10):

3) ____________________ **Daily / Weekly / Monthly**

Severity (0–10):

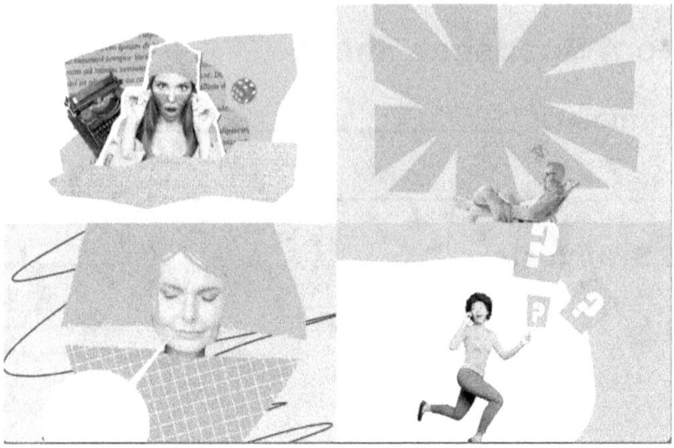

3. Patterns:

When did it/they start?

Any cycle triggers?

* * *

4. What I've Tried Already:

5. What Helps (even a little):

6. What Makes (Sh)It Worse:

7. Previous Dismissals I Want Addressed:

***8. What I Want From This Visit* (check all that apply):**

☐ Symptom relief strategies

☐ Medication options (stimulant, non-stimulant for ADHD in particular if not yet prescribed and others if interested)

☐ Non-HRT supplements

☐ MHT: I want an informed discussion about the latest research — not outdated fear based on 2002 data.

☐ Specialist referrals for neurobiological conditions and peri/menopause, as well as GAHT and other gender-affirming treatments if needed

☐ Lifestyle strategies discussion (nutrition/exercise/mental health)

☐ Documentation for workplace/school

☐ Hormone testing (if you still want it — see note on p. 72)

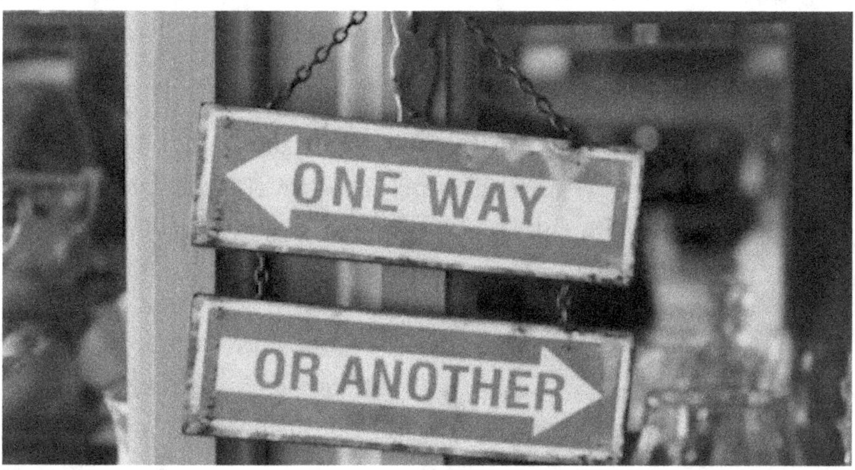

☐ Believe me. My symptoms are real. If you can't believe me, I'll find someone who will. Full stop.

See the Symptom Severity Decoder below for help rating your issues with a pinch of levity and dash of snark. Because laughter is medicine, too.

The Peri/Meno Neurodivergent Symptom Severity Decoder

A 1–10 scale for when your brain, body, and soul are on strike, but nobody handed you a picket sign. No softeners. Just raw and real descriptors for every level of WTF-your-body-is-doing.

1 – "Oh look, a mild inconvenience." You notice something's off, but you remember why you walked into the room. You make a joke. You almost feel guilty for even noticing. You'll pay for the arrogance of that self-assurance tomorrow.

2 – "That's new... but sure." You're mostly functioning but slightly suspicious of your own body. Something creaked or blinked or flared or quit, but hey, you've got shit to do. This is fine.

3 – "I could probably survive a dinner party like this... if no one asks me how I'm doing." Low-level emotional chaos. You're practicing facial expressions in case someone expects you to be coherent. You are *not* coherent.

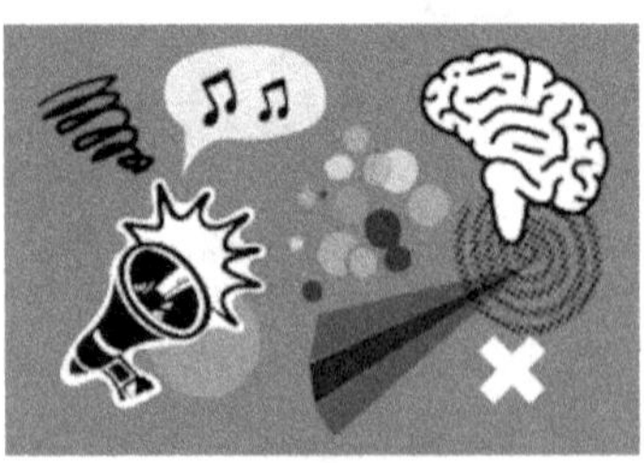

4 – "Is this sensory hell or just Target on a Saturday?" You're overstimulated by people and fluorescent lights. You're debating whether to scream, cry, or buy another notebook you'll never use. You do all three. And add a candy bar in the checkout aisle. Apparently four is the new "three's the charm."

5 – "Please tell my nervous system that we're not under attack!" Mid-tier malfunction. Your pain, fatigue, brain fog, and rage are all playing tug-of-war with your executive function. You're the rope.

6 – "Unclear if this is perimenopause or I'm being hunted for sport." You've cried in public, ghosted everyone, rage-cleaned everything, and now you're horizontal, wondering if you're allergic to gravity. Probably.

7 – "Do not touch me, talk to me, or ask me to fill out a form." Every cell is protesting. Your skin hurts. Your inbox hurts. Your name hurts. This is a full-on sensory-emotional hostage situation. Blink once if you're still technically alive.

8 – "I have achieved maximum volatility. Approach at your own risk." You are deeply exhausted and violently awake. You might break something. Maybe a chair. Maybe a belief system.

9 – "There is no 'before.' There is only this." You are dissociating while arguing with the pharmacy while leaking tears while doing eight mental checklists that go nowhere. Your executive dysfunction is mocking you.

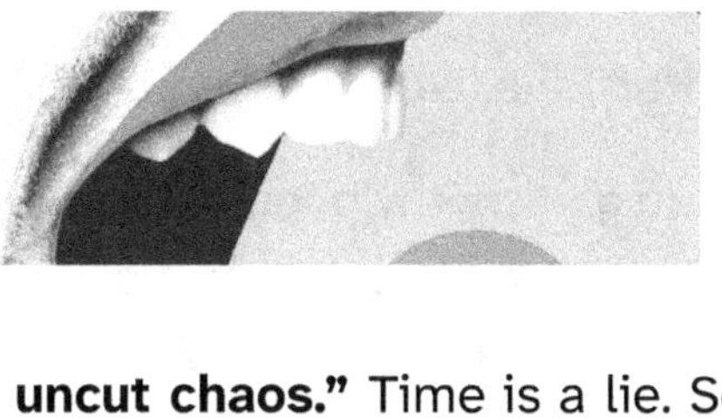

10 – "I am pure, uncut chaos." Time is a lie. So is the doctor. In a state of full-body primal scream, you're made entirely of hot flashes and vengeance. You are the final boss.

The Truth About Hormone Testing

Hormone tests *seem* like the obvious answer. But the reality?

Hormone levels fluctuate wildly — even within a day — making most one-time tests unreliable for diagnosing perimenopause.

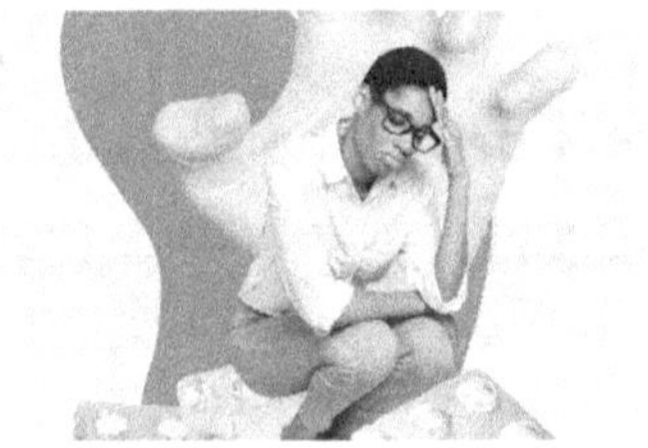

Diagnosis should come from symptoms + history, which are better indicators than a one-time blood draw (Santoro & Neal-Perry 2024). *Know this: "normal" labs don't erase your lived experience.*

Don't let a "normal" result convince you your symptoms aren't real.

A note about Stimulant & Non-Stimulant ADHD Meds in Context

Are ADHD meds worth it? And do I have options?

Yes — stimulant medications are the gold standard for adults with ADHD when it comes to improving attention, executive function, and daily life management. But treatment is not one-size-fits-all.

Stimulants = First-Line, But It's Personal

- Stimulants (e.g., methylphenidate, amphetamines) are approved as the first-choice medications for adult ADHD by guidelines from AADPA and CDC (2024), with a strong evidence base in randomized controlled trials.

• Meta-analysis confirms stimulants *strongly reduce* core ADHD symptoms and improve executive function across adult cohorts.

Non-Stimulants = Valid & Valuable

• Non-stimulants (like atomoxetine, guanfacine, viloxazine) are FDA-approved alternatives and are recommended for those who can't tolerate stimulants or have contraindications.

• They can be used alone or in combination and have less potential for misuse.

Individualized Treatment Planning

Every medication plan is unique — tailored to your body, existing conditions, allergies, sensitivities, and other meds you're already taking. It's about finding what works *for you.*

Summary:

- Stimulants are the fastest acting and most studied, but effective non-stimulants exist as well.
- Coaching plus therapy are critical support pillars.

None of this is optional — it's about designing a treatment ecosystem around you, customized to support your individual and unique needs.

Hormone Replacement Therapy: The Facts

In 2002, the **WHI study** scared millions by claiming HRT (or MHT, as we've referred to it here per the current terminology) significantly increased cancer and heart disease risk. That data has since been **retracted and clarified**:

• The hormones used in this study were **synthetic**. Bioidentical (or body identical) hormones commonly used now have a molecular structure that is identical to the hormones our bodies naturally produce (ACOG, 2023). Also, because they are **chemically identical,** they are easily absorbed, decreasing the potential for side effects. Always consult a medical provider.

• When used properly (especially in your 40s or early 50s), bioidentical **estrogen and progesterone** are safe and often beneficial. Nevertheless, controversy still looms around age at initiation, route of administration, and formulation.

• NAMS (2024) and ACOG (2023) now endorse MHT as the ***most effective treatment for menopausal symptoms***, with benefits often outweighing risks for most AFAB people under 60, with many cis women over 60 now using MHT as well.

• **Insertable genital estradiol** can be life-changing for dryness and painful intimacy. If you are experiencing discomfort, you may be a candidate this. Again, consult your provider.

• **Testosterone therapy** may be appropriate for some, particularly for libido, muscle, and mood. While it is not currently FDA-approved for women in the US, **testosterone is not just a "male hormone,"** no matter how much bad science and cultural nonsense try to sell that lie. It plays **a vital role** in the health of all people dealing with hormonal shifts. A recent retrospective observational study suggests that individualized testosterone therapy may help more than libido, including mood, energy, cognition, and depression (Elggren et al., 2026). Anecdotal evidence is a start, but not enough. Consult your provider for potential treatments.

Nuance Alert: Neurodivergent Brains Need Customized Care

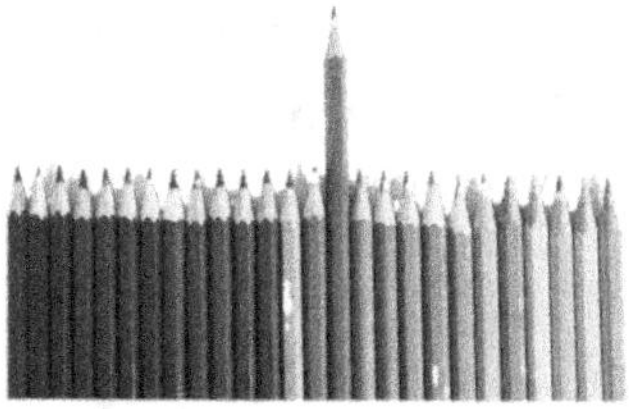

Most ADHD and MHT protocols were developed and tested primarily in neurotypical populations. Unfortunately, there's still very limited research on how these treatments work — or don't — for neurodivergent cis women, let alone trans men and genderqueer people during perimenopause. Here's what we know regarding cisgender women:

Research shows that **hormonal fluctuations** (like estrogen decline in perimenopause) can **alter** how stimulant meds are absorbed and processed—sometimes reducing their effectiveness just when ND brains need clarity most.

For instance, some women with ADHD report needing a **slightly higher medication dose** during low-estrogen phases such as premenstrual weeks or during perimenopause.

Similarly, standard MHT regimens may not fit ND bodies. Preliminary data suggests **neurodivergent cis women** (e.g., ADHD, autistic) are **more sensitive to hormone dosage and delivery method** — and may do better with body-identical, transdermal options to avoid mood swings and overstimulation.

In contrast, some ND folks **may not tolerate bioidentical progesterone** and may feel best with a synthetic option. And, some ND women report major sensitivities to MHT in general.

Again, we can't stress enough, **there is no one-size-fits-all**. Just because stimulant medication may be considered the gold standard treatment for ADHD in the same way that HRT is considered the safest and most effective treatment for peri/menopausal symptoms and hormone decline doesn't mean that you have to take one, the other, or both. **Stimulants may not be the best option** for you if you are **Autistic and/or OCD**, for example. And if you are a **breast cancer survivor** or have the gene and take **estrogen blockers**, standard MHT may not be appropriate for you.

Still, the right question isn't "can I take MHT?," only to get a Yes/No response, but rather "what are the specific risks and benefits for ME?" The fact is, this isn't your provider's choice: it's actually yours. "No" isn't always the safest choice, but rather a choice with a different set of risks.

BOTTOM LINE: ***You know your body + brain best.***

Treatments aren't one-size-fits-all. Your neurodivergent brain + race/ethnicity + gender identity + hormonal shifts = a unique response.

You deserve a treatment plan designed for your brain and body —especially during perimenopause. ***Be your own advocate****: if something is off, push for adjustments or second opinions until it feels right.*

Fill-in-the-Blank Script for Provider Visits

(Grab this from the printables folder ... QR code on pp. 24 & 38 ... or write directly in this book and take it with you.)

Hi. I'm here because my daily life is being significantly disrupted by symptoms I believe are connected to peri-menopause (hormonal shifts) and/or neurodivergence.

Here are the three main symptoms disrupting my life:

1.

2.

3.

I've been tracking them. Here are the patterns I've noticed:

____

____

____

____

____

I'd like us to focus today on exploring:

☐ Symptom relief

☐ Medications (stimulant or non-stimulant)

☐ Non-MHT supplements

☐ MHT (please discuss latest evidence)

☐ Specialist Referrals (Neuroaffirming care, Menopause/Hormone care, Gender-affirming care)

☐ Documentation

☐ Lifestyle strategies

☐ Hormone testing (if indicated)

And most importantly: Believe me when I say my symptoms are real.

* * *

☑ Appointment Prep Checklist

☐ **Print & bring your Symptom Snapshot**

☐ **Highlight your top 1–2 priorities**

☐ **Bring a support person or ask to record the visit**

☐ **Rehearse your provider script**

☐ **Write down follow-up steps before leaving**

☐ **If dismissed: Find another provider.**

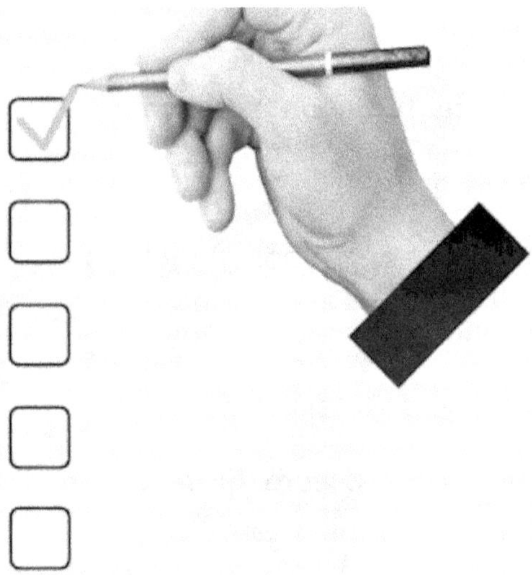

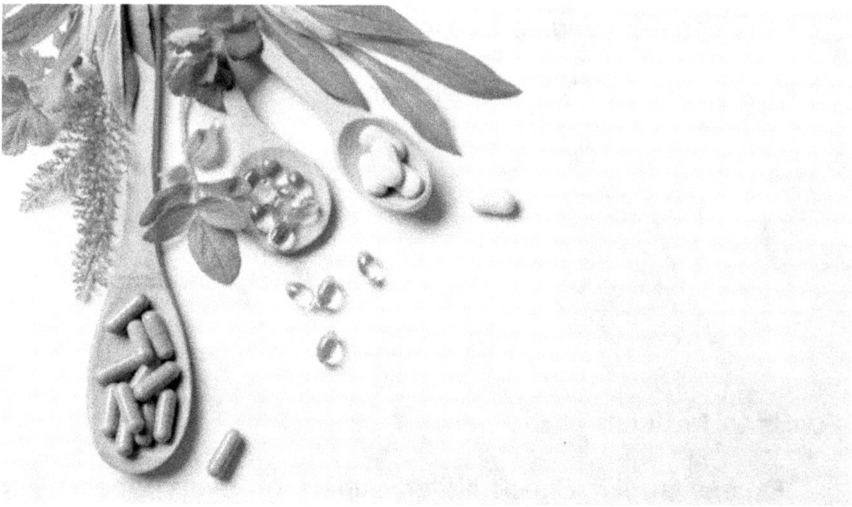

Food, Inflammation & Self-Compassion: Non-MHT Supplements & Nutrition Guide

Evidence-Based Non-MHT Supplements (not medical advice: as always, consult your providers before starting anything new)

✔ Omega-3 fatty acids → Reduce inflammation & hot flashes

✔ Black cohosh → Some support for hot flashes & mood

✔ Vitamin D & calcium → Bone health, mood

✔ Magnesium glycinate → Sleep, anxiety, muscle calm

✔ B-Complex → Energy & cognitive support

Eat to fight inflammation & nourish your nervous system.

Foods to Prioritize:

☑ Colorful fruits & vegetables ☑ Whole grains

☑ Fatty fish — *or vegetarian*: flaxseed, chia, walnuts, sea-weed

☑ Olive oil & nuts ☑ Turmeric, ginger

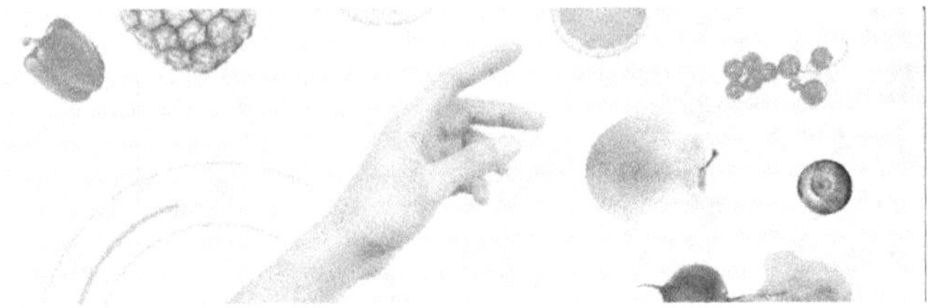

Foods to Reduce:

🚫 **Excess sugar**: Check added sugars on every label; try to avoid added sugar whenever possible.

🚫 **Processed meats** (sorry, cold cuts, even plant-based)**:** too much added salt, among other things!

🚫 **Alcohol** (it's a sleep-wrecker, sorry wine): Wine, we still love you, but you don't seem to love us much anymore. You interfere with our sleep, and tbh, you just don't pair well with any medications we might be on...

Ultimately, all things in moderation. Now more than ever, it's good to be intentional with nutrition, but we should enjoy life. Tracking micro and macro nutrients can reveal significant gaps and/or possible toxicity-inducing overloads. It's not about restricting calories though. Fuck diets. And perfection. Eating something is better than eating nothing.

Track your intake if you want — Apps to Track Nutrition: Cronometer (free, upgrade for $5/mo if you want). But beware the optimization trap. The pursuit of perfection is futile, and frankly, flawed and no fun.

Remember: It's not about restriction — it's about support.

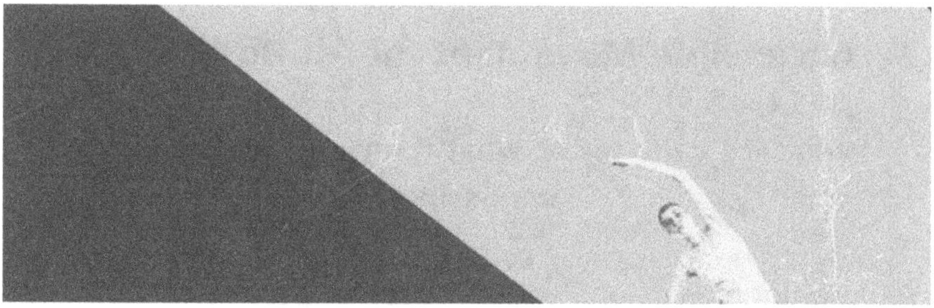

Movement Is Medicine

You don't need to punish your body. You don't need to earn your rest. You just need to move — regularly & kindly.

Your 5-Minute Victory Circuit:

✔ 60 seconds: Sun salutations

✔ 60 seconds: Jumping jacks

✔ 60 seconds: Plank (on knees if needed)

✔ 60 seconds: Weighted squats or wall sit

✔ 60 seconds: Stretch & breathe

And if nothing else? Go outside & walk. You don't have to run. You don't have to power walk. You don't have to do 10,000 steps. No marathons required. Even 10 minutes a day improves mood, stress, energy, sleep, bones, heart & brain (and you'll probably curse less at strangers).

That's a win. I know you know this! You got this!

🪑 Accessible Movement for All Bodies

"What if I can't walk? What if my pain makes moving impossible?"

You are not broken, and you still deserve the benefits of movement. Even small, seated or lying-down movements can help improve circulation, mood, energy, and reduce pain over time (Fong et al., 2016; Rimmer et al., 2021).

Here's a **5-Minute Chair Victory Routine**, adapted from the CDC & Arthritis Foundation recommendations:

🪑 5-Minute Chair Victory Routine

(Do each for ~1 minute — seated in a sturdy chair with feet flat on the floor. Stop if you feel sharp pain.)

✅ **1. Seated Marching** — Lift one knee, then the other, like you're marching in place — Option: Pump your arms gently

✅ **2. Seated Side Twists** — Place hands on hips or cross arms — Slowly twist upper body side to side — Feel your waist & spine gently stretch

✅ **3. Seated Jumping Jacks (Arms Only)** — Start with hands at your sides — Bring arms overhead like a jumping jack & back down — Keep feet still

✅ **4. Shoulder Rolls** — Roll shoulders forward & back in big, slow circles

✅ **5. Seated Leg Extensions** — Straighten one leg & hold for 3–5 seconds, then switch — Engage thigh muscles

Even 5 minutes of gentle seated movement can improve circulation, ease stiffness, and release mood-lifting endorphins. You don't have to be pain-free or able to stand to benefit.

***And remember:* Rest is productive:** Micro-naps (10–20 min) restore focus, memory, and regulate mood (Sood et al., 2019).

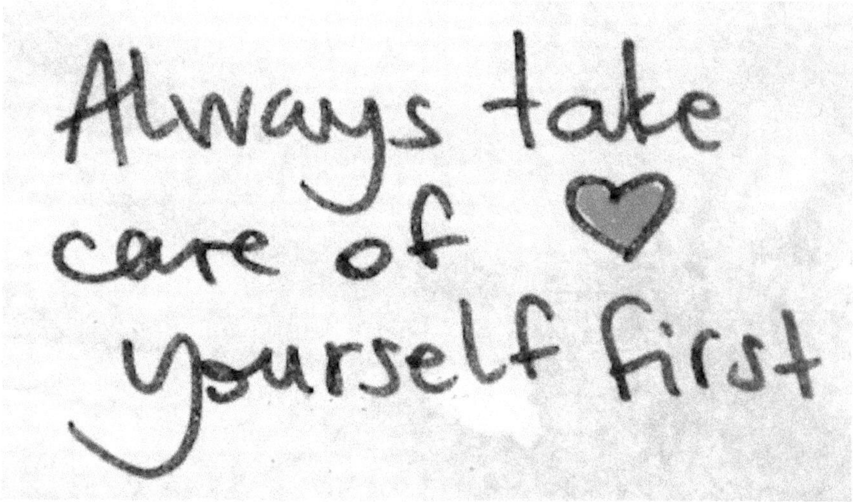

💜 Closing & Encouragement

You deserve care. And if you're dismissed? Leave.

Find a provider who respects you.

As we move into executive function rescue strategies in the next chapter, keep in mind that no one expects you to navigate these challenges without help. The right providers can lighten the load and help you thrive in midlife's most demanding moments.

Chapter 3

Executive Function Rescue

Theme: Momentum

Goal: Help you unjam your overwhelmed brain and take small, meaningful actions — even when hormones and executive dysfunction team up against you.

* * *

Trying to get your shit together when your hormones are rioting and your neurotransmitters have called in sick is not a failure.

It's biology. And here's how to outsmart it anyway.

Why It's Not 'Just You Losing It'

Newer studies show that fluctuating estrogen directly impacts working memory, attention, and overall executive function—areas already challenged in neurodivergent brains (Kooij et al., 2025; Luine, 2014; Russell et al., 2019). This explains why planning, prioritizing, and following through can feel exponentially harder now.

The latest data also suggests that stimulant medications, while still the gold standard for ADHD, may work differently during these hormonal shifts, requiring dose adjustments or complementary support strategies (ADDitude, 2024; Epperson et al., 2015). This chapter arms you with realistic strategies—and permission to lower the bar—so you can regain momentum.

What You'll Find in Chapter 3:

☑ **Daily Dopamine Planner**

☑ **Mini-Mission Cards**

☑ **Sensory Overload Rescue Kit**

☑ **Brain Break Cards**

☑ **Validation, science, and step-by-step strategies** to keep going even when your brain bails

Welcome & Why This Matters

Executive dysfunction: the fine art of wanting to do something, knowing it's important, even caring deeply about it ... and still not being able to start. Or finish. Or even remember what the hell you were supposed to do.

During perimenopause + neurodivergence, your brain's "manager" (the prefrontal cortex) is drunk, your dopamine tank is empty, and everything feels like too much.

Chapter 3 gives you:

✔ A way to unjam your brain

✔ Permission to do less

✔ Dopamine-friendly micro-plans

✔ Sensory-friendly SOS strategies

✔ Tiny wins to build momentum without the shame spiral

Executive Dysfunction Explained

Your executive functions are like an overworked manager who controls:

☑ Planning & prioritizing

☑ Switching focus

☑ Emotion regulation

☑ Task initiation & follow-through

Hormonal chaos + neurodivergent wiring = that manager quits mid-shift and leaves you with a to-do list that feels like running a marathon in flip-flops. *It's not laziness.* **It's neurology.**

Note on ADHD Medications & Hormonal Shifts

Stimulant medications (such as methylphenidate and amphetamine-based options) remain the gold standard for treating ADHD because they target dopamine and norepinephrine pathways—boosting motivation, focus, and impulse control (Bidwell et al., 2011; Epperson et al., 2015; Shanmugan et al., 2017).

But here's the nuance no one tells us: hormonal changes during perimenopause and menopause can change how these medications work in your body. You may notice shifts in effectiveness or side effects as your estrogen and progesterone levels fluctuate (Kooij et al., 2025).

Treatment plans must be individualized. If you're finding your medication isn't working like it used to, it doesn't mean you're "failing treatment"— it means your brain and body need adjustments. Partner with a provider who *gets it* to revisit your dose, timing, or consider non-stimulant medications if needed. ADHD coaches and therapists who specialize in neurodivergence can also be invaluable in building supportive strategies around any medication plan.

Estrogen Fluctuations: *Why Hormones Wreck Your Working Memory*

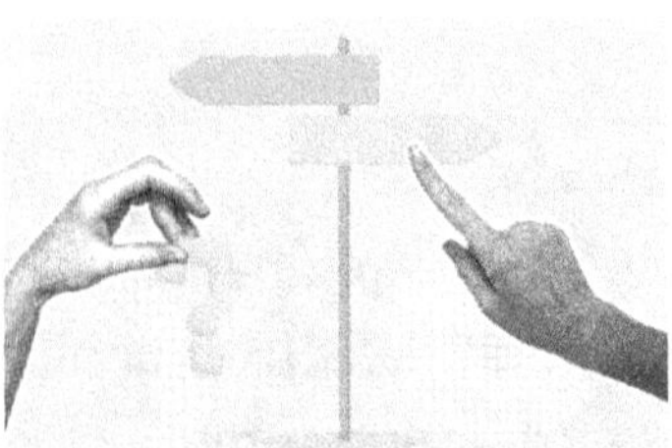

Working memory (your brain's mental Post-It note) and executive function are particularly sensitive to estrogen fluctuations. Research shows that as estrogen drops, we experience reduced synaptic plasticity and weaker prefrontal cortex activation—aka the parts of the brain responsible for planning, prioritizing, and remembering why you walked into the kitchen (Luine, 2014; Russell et al., 2019).

Kooij et al.'s position paper on the current research confirms that for neurodivergent AFAB people, these shifts can feel even more intense. Knowing this isn't a character flaw can help you respond with compassion—and get the right support.

⚡ Quickstart Instructions

1 **Pick *one* task** from the Daily Dopamine Planner.

2 **Break it down** with a Mini-Mission Card.

3 **Keep the Brain Break Cards handy** for when you freeze.

4 **Use the Sensory Overload Rescue Kit** when your environment feels like it's attacking you.

First, a story...

Perpetually Thirty Minutes Behind (with Olympic Gold Consistency)

I have a long, (un)decorated history of being late. Late to parties (I arrive just in time for the good-bye hugs ... don't get me started on leaving without saying goodbye ... yes, I've done it ... a lot).

Late getting my kids to soccer/gymnastics/the dentist, you-name-it because a water bottle hid under the couch and the uniform was "mysteriously" inside a pillowcase. My kids were late for school so much (sometimes on them, but often because of me) that the social worker at my daughter's school knew us by name and on sight. Late leaving for beach vacations—car packed, snacks ready, and me sprinting back inside ten times for the 'right' sunscreen, chargers, to clean the bathroom sink, and yet still actually forgot my swimsuits one year.

Speaking of packing for trips (slight tangent, but whatever, I have ADHD), once when I was a professor, I went to Spain for a conference, and I literally forgot to pack. I wish I were kidding. When I arrived at my hotel room in Madrid and opened my suitcase, I realized that all I'd packed were socks and underwear. I was stuck wearing the same jeans, blouse, jacket and boots I wore on the plane for the next three days. It was humiliating. I was so disappointed and angry with myself.

OK, back to our regularly scheduled programming about lateness ...

My daughter and I almost missed a flight once and they were last calling our names over the PA system in the airport as we exited security, and I just remember yelling frantically, RUN! Which we did and made it to the gate right as they were about to close it.

I was also often late to my own classes. Sigh. Yes. A student once wrote in a scathing end-of-semester evaluation: "It's hard to learn punctuality from someone who treats time like a suggestion." Fair.

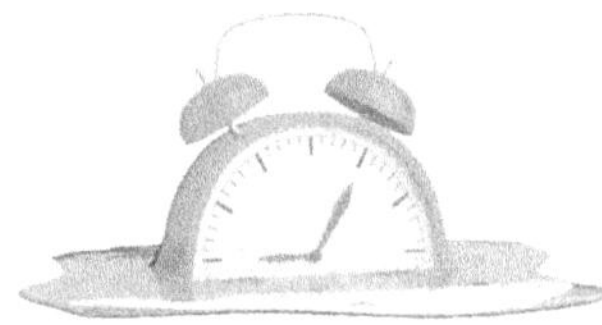

More recently, after my ADHD diagnosis, some skills slid backward in that strange way they do when awareness outruns systems. Bills? Late. Interest and penalties? Paid—with feeling. Doctor's appointments? A scavenger hunt where the final clue is me, breathless, at the wrong building.

For years, lateness felt like proof I was an incompetent adult cosplaying responsibility. Being late, causing others to be late, and inconveniencing people is embarrassing, and it sends a message that you don't respect their time. And frankly, that's just not cool. But I'm not alone. I'm not broken. I finally have language for what's happening: executive (dys)function—the optimistic time math, the task-switching tolls, the leaving-the-house obstacle course. Layer midlife hormones on top (hello, fog, fatigue, and emotional static), and the margins vanish.

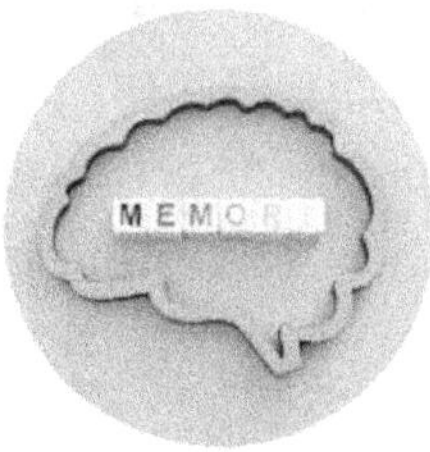

Knowing this changes the story. Now I plan for "transition time" like it's an actual task. I front-load the boring steps when my brain has gas in the tank. I use alarms that are embarrassingly early, keep a "go bag," and set due dates a day —ok, fine, two to three days—ahead. Most importantly, I work with my brain, not against it. I still run late sometimes. But now it's with compassion, better tools, and a quiet confidence that I can build a life that fits the wiring I have—not the schedule I wish I kept.

The Modular Task Toolkit: "Doom Pile" Crushers for Every Day

When energy dips or brain fog rolls in, the doom pile grows larger, and shame grows with it. You may look around and see not just clutter, but evidence of every plan that fell apart. For neurodivergent adults in midlife, this feels like a daily reminder that the world expects a type of order your mind and body refuse to produce. The doom pile has roots in more than just forgetfulness—it's born from mental overload, unpredictable motivation, and the constant effort to keep up with demands that outpace your resources.

To counter this, try a modular approach—a toolkit that meets you where you are, letting you mix and match supports as needed. The toolkit's core idea is flexibility: tasks can be split, swapped, or scaled down depending on your day's capacity.

Start with the timer method. Set a kitchen timer or your phone for five minutes and focus on just one area—the mail stack, the laundry chair, the paper pile by the door. When the timer rings, stop. If energy remains, set it again. If not, step away guilt-free. This method allows you to break inertia and build momentum without demanding perfection or completion.

Next, try "mini-mission" task cards. Write one simple action per card—"put three things in the trash," "shred old receipts," "fold five shirts." Place these cards where you see the doom pile most often. On hard days, pick a single card and complete just that tiny task. Each finished card represents progress, regardless of the pile's remaining size. For those who thrive on external cues, create a "doom pile playlist"—music or podcasts that make chores less dull and transform cleaning into a less isolating experience. The playlist becomes a subtle cue for action; put it on whenever you face your pile.

Micro-tasking is your ally. There is no rule that says chores must be completed all at once. Fold socks today and leave shirts for tomorrow. Open just one envelope instead of the entire mail stack. Wipe one countertop rather than cleaning the whole kitchen. Allowing yourself to do small pieces at a time relieves pressure and chips away at shame. You are not failing by leaving things unfinished; you are adapting to the real limits of executive function and hormonal ups and downs.

Shame thrives when tasks appear unmanageable and progress feels invisible. Counter this by making completion visible, no matter how small the step. **Use a "done jar"**—every time you finish a card or micro-task, drop a token or slip of paper inside. Over time, the jar fills up, creating a tangible record of effort and accomplishment that fights back against self-criticism.

Some find it helpful to display finished task cards on a cork board or wall as a visual reminder that tasks were handled, even if not all at once.

Accountability and rewards may help shift motivation from dread to encouragement. Pair up with someone you trust—a friend, partner, or online buddy—and agree to check in after each micro-task session. Share photos or text updates: "I cleared one corner today," "Two more bills opened." Celebrate each other's wins with kind words or emoji reactions; validation from another person can cut through isolation and reinforce progress. If you live with others, invite them to join in—task-sharing turns chores into brief moments of connection rather than solo battles.

Every modular tool in this toolkit has one purpose: to bring tasks back into reach and remind you that progress counts even when it doesn't look like what others expect.

The doom pile may never disappear completely; it will expand and contract as life shifts. But with mix-and-match supports, visual reminders of progress, accountability partners, and genuine rewards, you can keep chaos from ruling your space or self-worth. Each card turned over or token dropped in the jar matters—a quiet act of resistance against the myth that only perfect completion deserves pride. Screw that!

Daily Dopamine Planner

What counts as a "Big Priority"?

Your "big priority" doesn't have to be something monumental. It's simply the **most important thing** you'd like **to move**

forward today. It could be sending one email you've been avoiding, doing a load of laundry, or calling the pharmacy.

Your Big Priority is essentially **ONE task that**, if it gets done today, **will make you feel a little lighter** — like you showed up for yourself. That's it. **It should be simple** enough that it can stand on its own, *or* you identify the micro-tasks it's made of.

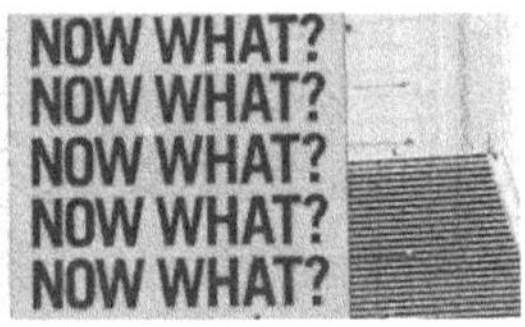

And remember: **rest can be a priority.** If your body is asking for downtime, it's valid to list "rest" as your big focus for the day.

Examples of Big Priorities:

✔ Make & eat breakfast

✔ Text doctor's office to book appointment

✔ Put away laundry from yesterday (or last month, in my case)

✔ Empty/load the dishwasher

✔ Pay one bill online

✔ Take a walk outside for 10 minutes

✔ Rest deliberately (yes — "nap" can be your Big Priority!)

If you find yourself frozen because the Big Priority seems too big:

PAUSE. — Ask yourself: "Are there micro-tasks involved? If yes, what are they? **Write them down** as mini-missions below. Or conversely, maybe those micro-tasks need to be their own "big priorities."

It's your body and brain, and the goal is to preserve your bandwidth shame-free. When life feels too much, you don't need to do everything. You can do *one* thing — broken down into baby steps.

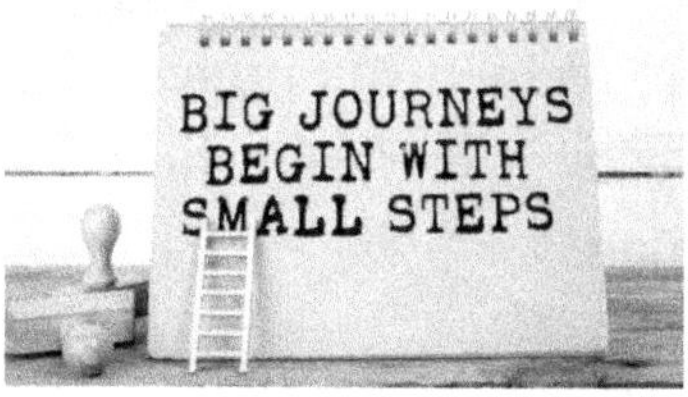

MINI-MISSION (TASK):

Task 1- (less than 5 minutes)

Task 2- (less than 5 minutes)

Task 3- (less than 5 minutes)

REWARD

Head to your printables folder Online to grab these cards.

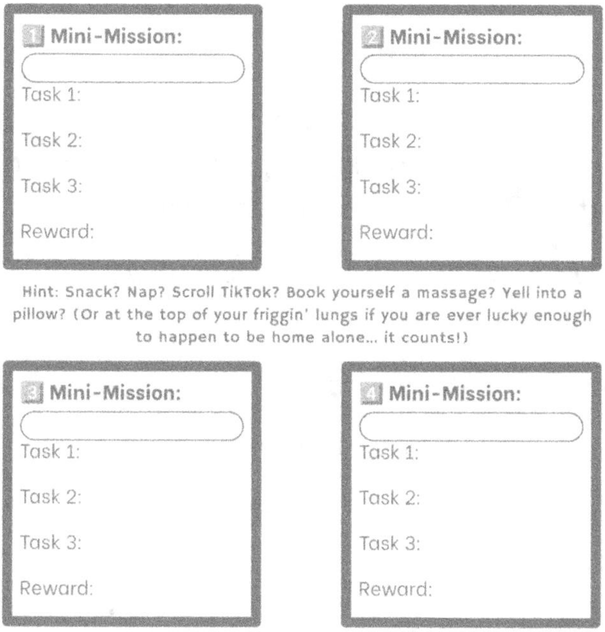
1 Mini-Mission:
Task 1:
Task 2:
Task 3:
Reward:

2 Mini-Mission:
Task 1:
Task 2:
Task 3:
Reward:

Hint: Snack? Nap? Scroll TikTok? Book yourself a massage? Yell into a pillow? (Or at the top of your friggin' lungs if you are ever lucky enough to happen to be home alone... it counts!)

3 Mini-Mission:
Task 1:
Task 2:
Task 3:
Reward:

4 Mini-Mission:
Task 1:
Task 2:
Task 3:
Reward:

Evening Reflection: "What Actually Got Done?"

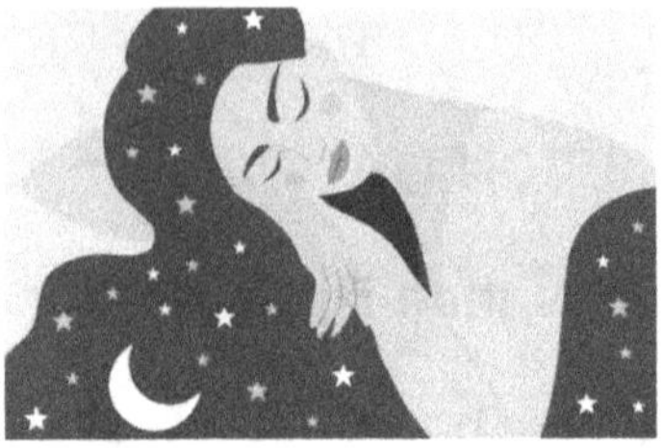

The "What Actually Got Done?" section is not here to shame you — it's here to help you notice what you *did*, even if it wasn't the thing you planned.

Did you brush your teeth?

Did you drink water?

Did you rest?

Did you just survive the day?

Those count. You count. Write them down.

Rest = A Legitimate Priority

You are not broken for needing rest — you're human. Intentional rest restores executive function, improves memory, reduces stress hormones, and makes you more capable tomorrow.

Even micro-naps — short naps of 10–20 minutes — are scientifically shown to:

✔ Improve mood & alertness

✔ Boost memory consolidation

✔ Reduce fatigue without grogginess (Mednick et al., 2002; Faraut et al., 2015)

* * *

Suggested Micro-Rest Ideas:

- Lie down & close your eyes for 10 minutes

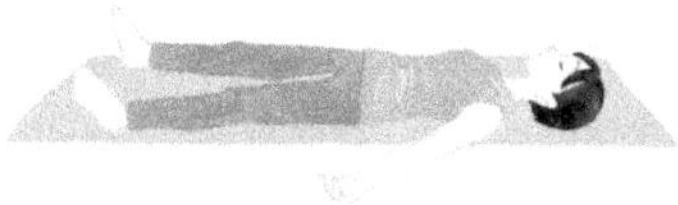

- Sit in a quiet room & listen to calming music
- Sit outside & stare at clouds
- Turn off your phone for 15 minutes & breathe

You don't need to earn rest — you already deserve it.

Planner Layout (example):

Morning:

Big Priority (examples: empty dishwasher, walk, nap):

____

Does this priority have micro-tasks?

□ No → go do it

□ Yes → list here:

1- ____________________

2- ____________________

3- ____________________

Three (or fewer) Mini Tasks

1- ____________________

2- ____________________

3- ____________________

Evening:

What Actually Got Done?

(Even if it's: "I cried and brushed my teeth. Still counts.")

Something You're Proud Of?

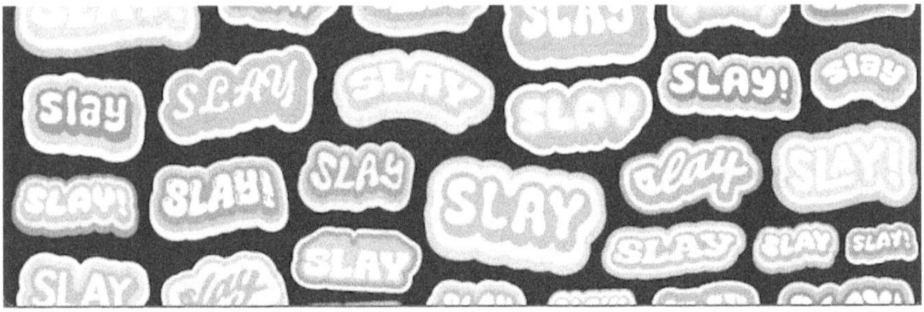

This planner is in your printables toolkit Online.

(QR code on p. 24 & 38)

* * *

Sensory-Friendly Home Hacks for Hot Flashes & Overwhelm

Your home should offer relief, yet for many neurodivergent adults in midlife, it often becomes a battleground of sensory triggers. With menopause, the threshold for overload can shrink further. Suddenly, what used to be a minor annoyance—like a synthetic pillowcase or the whir of an appliance—can trigger discomfort, agitation, or even a full shutdown.

Clothing and fabric choices matter more than ever as tactile sensitivity can spike with hormonal changes. Tagless shirts, seamless socks, and loose-fitting pants worn around the house can make the difference between comfort and distraction.

Temperature also tops the list: hot flashes are unpredictable and can turn your bedroom into a furnace at midnight. Synthetic bedding traps heat, making sleep elusive and rest incomplete. Swapping these out for natural, breathable fibers such as cotton or bamboo can reduce the sensation of being "stuck in your own skin." When it comes to bedding, choose materials with moisture-wicking properties and avoid heavy comforters that trap heat. Keep a lightweight robe or wrap by your bed to slip on during night sweats; changing textures quickly can reset your tactile system and help you return to sleep.

Keep a quiet, oscillating fan within reach—not just for cooling, but for steady white noise that soothes rather than irritates. For those who crave pressure, a weighted blanket made from cooling fabric blends can offer security without stifling warmth. Soft blankets or textured cushions on the couch provide tactile comfort and grounding when emotions run high.

Lighting causes more harm than many realize. Overhead lights, especially those with a blue or harsh white tone, can make sensory sensitivity worse and spark headaches. Replace bulbs with softer, warm-toned LEDs or consider floor and table lamps with dimming options. If flickering from old fixtures is an issue (often missed by neurotypical partners), swapping to newer bulbs or using lampshades can reduce eye strain.

For late-night comfort or early mornings, a salt lamp or softly shaded nightlight can help you navigate without a jolt to your system. Noise is another hidden adversary. **Sounds intensify during hormonal shifts**; the kitchen clatter, children's voices, or traffic become almost unbearable. Invest in well-cushioned noise-canceling headphones or soft silicone earplugs for those chaotic hours when your nervous system needs shelter.

If you share space, communicate your needs to others—let them know there will be times when you need silence to recover.

No home is too small for a sensory safe zone—a designated area for retreat and regulation when overwhelm hits hard. Even a single chair in the quietest corner can become your sanctuary. Choose a space with soft lighting and minimal clutter; add a favorite throw or weighted lap pad for instant comfort. Place fidget toys, textured objects, or sensory stones within arm's reach to occupy restless hands and redirect anxious energy. If possible, include an air purifier or essential oil diffuser with calming scents like lavender or cedarwood. **This safe zone is not selfish; it is vital for recovery and emotional stability.**

For those times when everything feels "too much," having a simple cheat sheet can make self-regulation easier.

On the refrigerator, tack up a list:

When overwhelmed, try these five things first—

☐ 1) Drink cold water

☐ 2) Sit in your safe zone

☐ 3) Put on headphones or earplugs

☐ 4) Change into soft clothes

☐ 5) Dim the lights or close blackout curtains.

Keep a "sensory reset basket" stocked with essentials—cooling wipes, a favorite snack, fidget tools, a small fan, and a soothing scented spray. Place it where you spend most of your time so you can access it quickly without searching.

Quick-Reference Checklist: Sensory Reset Basket

☐ Cooling face or body wipes ☐ Compact handheld fan

☐ Lightweight scarf or wrap ☐ Fidget toy (putty, ring, stone)

... I love my spinner rings ... people just think I'm accessorizing and that it's a style thing, unaware that these rings actually play an integral role in my sensory regulation.

☐ Noise-canceling headphones or silicone earplugs

☐ Soft eye mask ☐ Lavender or peppermint roller

☐ Favorite snack (easy to eat + comforting) ☐ Bottle of water

These modifications need not cost much or demand major renovations. The goal is to lower the barrier to comfort, so you can respond quickly when distress rises. Even small changes—

like moving a lamp or keeping headphones within reach—can shift your environment from hostile to healing. Remember that your brain's needs fluctuate; having flexible options on hand means you're ready to support yourself on even the most unpredictable days. Small adjustments add up, restoring both peace and control when sensory overload threatens to take over your home life.

Sensory Overload Rescue Mini-Kit

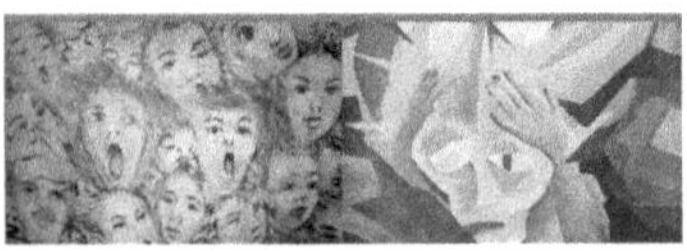

When the world feels too loud, too bright, too tight — this is your lifeline.

If It's Too Bright:

✔ Sunglasses

✔ Dim the lights

✔ Close your eyes

If It's Too Tight:

✔ Change into soft, loose clothes

✔ Weighted blanket

✔ Run cool water over your hands

If It's Too Much Emotionally:

✔ Box breathing (inhale 4, hold 4, exhale 4, hold 4)

✔ 5-4-3-2-1 grounding (name 5 things you see, 4 you feel, etc.)

✔ Step outside — even if just onto your porch.

Brain Break Cards

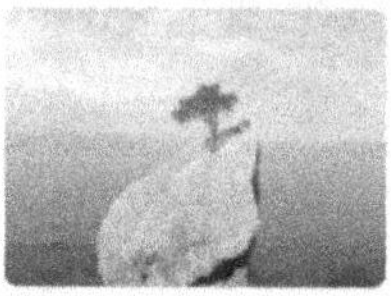

Stop scrolling.

Breathe for 60 seconds.

→ Your brain needs oxygen more than Instagram.

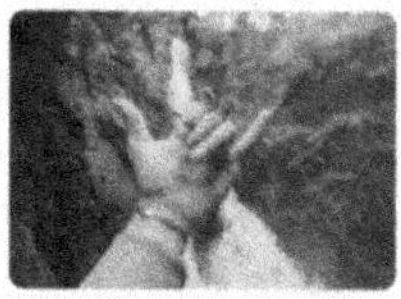

Loosen up.

Stand up and stretch.

***

→ Your body moves, your brain follows.

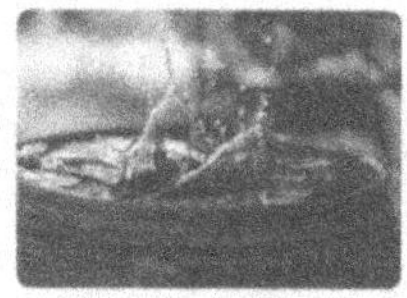

Hydrate.

Drink a glass of water.

***

→ Hydration is underrated and free.

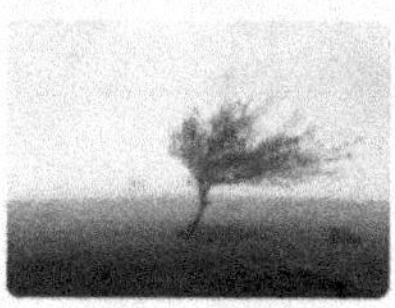

Simplify.

Write down ONE next step.

***

→ You don't need the whole plan yet.

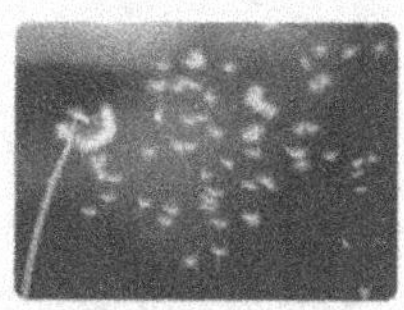

Shift.

Move something — even just your hands.

***

→ Stuck energy needs an exit.

When you're stuck and spiraling, grab one of these and reset. They're in your Online toolbox of printables.

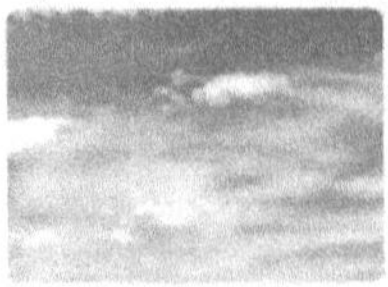

Slow down.

Step outside & look at the sky.

→ You are not the same size as your inbox.

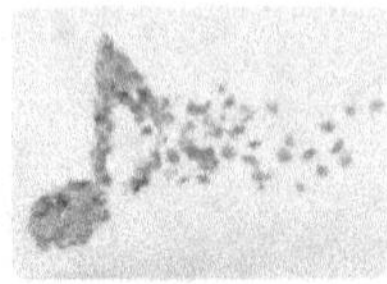

Listen.

Play a song you love.

***

→ Dopamine on demand.

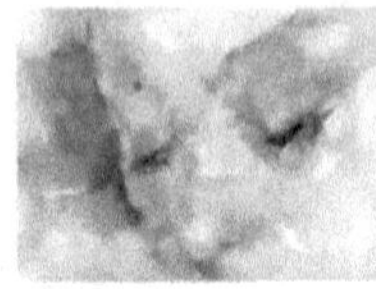

Relax.

Close your eyes for 2 minutes.

***

→ Micro-rest counts.

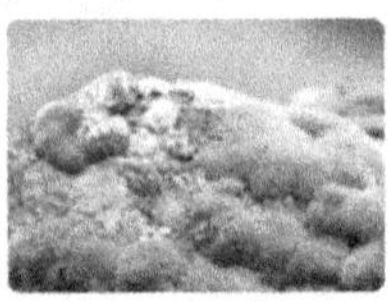

Connect.

Touch something soft or grounding.

***

→ Bring your senses back home.

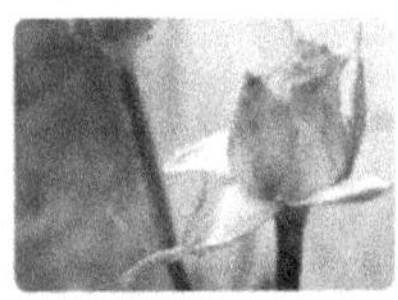

Lower the bar.

Tell yourself: I don't have to finish this perfectly.

Just start.

* * *

* * *

* * *

💗 Closing & Encouragement

You don't need to magically fix your brain. You don't need to be perfectly organized or productive. You just need a path through the overwhelm — one tiny win at a time. Executive function isn't broken beyond repair. It's just out of gas.

Refuel it. Support it. Celebrate even the smallest forward step.

Chapter 4

Reclaim Your Sleep

Theme: Restoration

Goal: Help you repair your wrecked sleep — without shame, without rigid rules, and without pretending that ND + hormones = 8 perfect hours.

* * *

Sleep Deprivation Is Not A Character Flaw.

Hormonal fluctuations don't just cause hot flashes—they disrupt the very systems that regulate sleep cycles, leading to chronic insomnia, anxiety, and "tornado brain" at night (Weber et al., 2014; Kooij et al., 2025). ND brains are especially vulnerable because racing thoughts, sensory sensitivities, and executive dysfunction can create multiple barriers to rest.

Cutting-edge research shows that breaking the cycle of sleep deprivation requires both nervous system support and strategic behavioral tweaks—many of which we'll cover in this chapter.

This chapter helps you reclaim the rest your brain and body desperately need in order to start repairing your nervous system.

What You'll Find in Chapter 4:

☑ **Deep-Dive Symptom Decoder: Sleep Problems & ND Brains** — Spot the root causes of your insomnia and learn what's hormonal, what's ND, and what's "both, actually."

☑ **Sleep Sabotage Self-Audit Worksheet** — A worksheet for tracking your unique obstacles, patterns, and wins—no more blaming yourself for "bad sleep hygiene."

☑ **ND-Friendly Sleep Hacks & Rituals Reference Sheet** — Cut through the sleep advice BS and find what really works for neurodivergent midlifers experiencing peri/menopause symptoms.

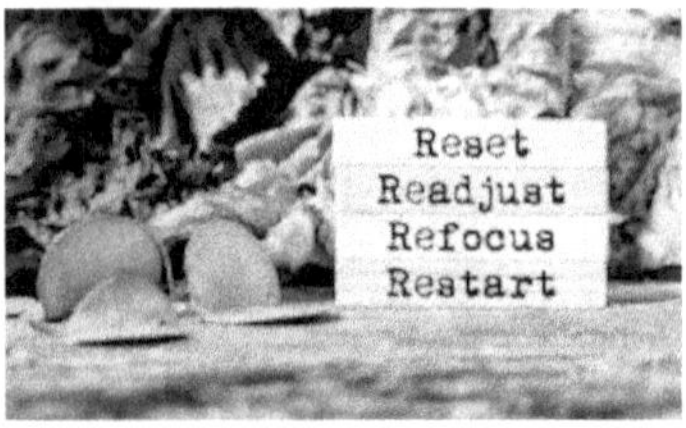

☑ **Reset Your Bedroom: Mini Declutter/Prep Guide** — Easy, actionable steps to make your sleep space work for your sensory needs.

☑ **Emergency Middle-of-the-Night Scripts & Self-Soothing Prompts** — When your brain's on fire at 3am, grab these scripts and get through the night with your sanity intact.

☑ **Partner Sleep Guide & Conversation Starters** — Ready-to-use prompts and scripts for explaining your sleep needs to your partner—without drama or shame.

☑ **White/Brown/Pink Noise App Recommendations**

Welcome & Why This Matters

Neurodivergence and menopause each screw with your sleep. Together? They throw an all-night rave in your nervous system and then blame you when you're exhausted.

You are not just "bad at sleeping." You're navigating estrogen withdrawal, cortisol spikes, and a brain that refuses to shut up.

We're not here to chase perfect sleep. We're here to stack wins — better quality rest, fewer shame spirals, and tools for the nights when sleep simply ... doesn't happen.

Why It Really Is Harder For ND Brains

If it feels like perimenopause & menopause hit you harder — that's because it does.

- ADHD and autism in particular are both associated with hyperarousal and delayed melatonin release.
- Estrogen decline directly disrupts REM sleep increases night wakings, and worsens mood.
- ND brains tend to catastrophize and struggle to "shut off," amplifying insomnia and exhaustion.

You're not imagining it: ND midlife brains create a perfect storm for wrecked nights. Add OCD's flood of intrusive thoughts as you lie down or chronic pain from hypermobility, for example, or [insert your other condition(s) here], and you quickly realize that a one-size-fits-all approach to sleep is impossible, and "perfect" sleep is a myth. You are neurocomplex, and that matters. You may need more nuanced care, but more than anything, you need self-compassion. This chapter aims to help you get rest back and stop blaming yourself when sleep doesn't look "normal."

Chapter 4 helps you:

✔ Reclaim the rest your brain and body desperately need

✔ Prioritize rest and sleep shame-free

✔ Strategize gentle nervous system repair in ways that don't feel invasive to your brain

⚡ **Quickstart Instructions**

1 **Read the ND Sleep Truths** to stop blaming yourself.

2 **Use the Sleep Symptom Decoder chart** to pinpoint what's really keeping you awake.

3 **Use the basic guide** to reset/declutter your bedroom.

4 **Choose one Wind-Down Ritual** to try tonight.

5 **Print and place the Emergency Insomnia Cards by your bed.**

6 **Try the 5-Minute Morning Reset tomorrow.**

7 **Initiate a conversation with your partner (if you have one) about sleep if applicable.** Use the note as a prompt. More on partners in chapter 5.

8 **Print the poster** in your Online toolbox. Frame it. Or don't. But place it somewhere where you'll see it everyday.

First, a story...

Living Half-Dead: Insomnia Didn't Kill Me, But It Tried

For twenty years, I lived on scraps of sleep. I'd lie in bed at 2 a.m. staring at the ceiling, wondering if maybe tonight would be the night my brain finally powered down. It never did. Doctors threw the whole pharmacy at me—Ambien, Lunesta, trazodone, benzos, even an antipsychotic meant for combat veterans. Nothing worked. Ambien didn't knock me out, but it sure knocked out my last shred of faith in medicine.

Running on fumes became my baseline. I taught classes, raised kids, and pretended I was fine while my brain and body quietly unraveled. Sleep isn't just a wellness checkbox—it's the foundation. Without it, everything else crumbles.

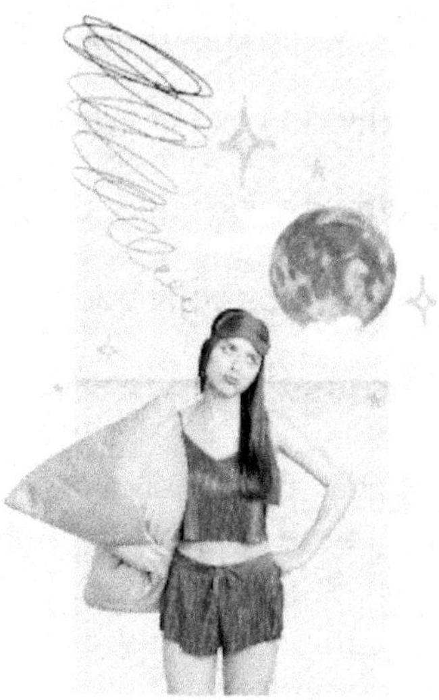

The breakthrough came only when I stopped treating symptoms and addressed the real wiring underneath. HRT helped stabilize my hormones, and when my doctor doubled my progesterone, I finally felt a shift. But the missing piece was ADHD treatment. Once I found the right stimulant dose, my tornado brain calmed enough to actually shut off at night. For the first time in decades, I slept like a human being, not a ghost in a haunted house.

It took me years of trial and error to get here, and that's the part nobody tells you: finding the right mix of meds and doses can be brutal. But it's worth enduring if you can, because the right treatment for *your* body and *your* brain is out there. Don't give up. Don't let anyone dismiss your exhaustion. Fight for your sleep like your life depends on it—because it does.

Remember: Rest — even imperfect — is medicine.

ND Sleep Truths Mini-Guide

1. Even resting quietly repairs tissues & lowers stress hormones.

2. ND brains have different circadian rhythms — your sleep window may simply be later.

3. Hormone shifts throw off your sleep architecture — it's real.

4. You don't need 8 perfect hours to function.

The ND + Hormone Sleep Saboteur Decoder

- Why do you lie awake even when you're exhausted?
- Why do you wake up every hour, or at 4:30 a.m. on the dot?
- Why does your body seem to conspire against rest?

Because sleep problems aren't just "one thing."

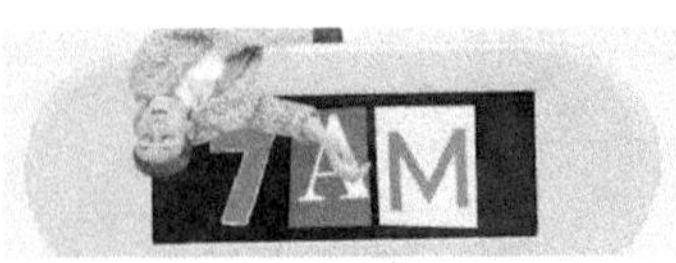

They're a tangled mess of hormones, neurotransmitters, and nervous system overdrive — especially in ND mid-lifers "blessed" with ovarian systems + a uterus at birth. Even if you don't have those anymore, you're not exempt from menopause or menopause-adjacent hormonal chaos. The following chart unpacks common sleep disruptions, their biological and neurological roots, and what they actually feel like. Because naming it is the first step to reclaiming it. It's in your toolbox, so print, circle or highlight symptoms you're experiencing if that helps.

Neuro-Hormonal Sleep Decoder

HIGHLIGHT OR CIRCLE YOUR SYMPTOMS

↓ = DECLINING, DECREASE IN, LOW *↑ = RISING, INCREASE IN, HIGH*

SYMPTOM	HORMONE/ NEURO-TRANSMITTER	WHAT'S GOING ON	WHAT IT FEELS LIKE
DIFFICULTY FALLING ASLEEP (MIND WON'T SHUT OFF)	↓ ESTROGEN + SUBSEQUENT DOPAMINE & PROGESTERONE ↑ CORTISOL	RACING THOUGHTS, HYPERFOCUS, INTRUSIVE WORRIES, MENTAL TO-DO LISTS THAT WON'T STOP	LYING IN THE DARK REPLAYING EVERY DECISION YOU MADE IN 1998, OR DESIGNING A NEW BUSINESS AT MIDNIGHT
WAKING UP REPEATEDLY	↓ ESTROGEN & PROGESTERONE + MELATONIN SUPPRESSION	SENSORY SENSITIVITY TO LIGHT/SOUND, LIGHT SLEEP PHASES, "ON-ALERT" NERVOUS SYSTEM	FEELING LIKE YOU NEVER HIT DEEP SLEEP; EVERY NOISE WAKES YOU; CLOCK-WATCHING
WAKING TOO EARLY & UNABLE TO FALL BACK ASLEEP	↓ ESTROGEN ↑ CORTISOL (IN THE MORNING)	ADHD TIME DYSMORPHIA + CATASTROPHIC THOUGHTS KICK IN AT DAWN	EYES SNAP OPEN AT 4:30AM WITH A SENSE OF PANIC OR DREAD
HOT FLASHES + NIGHT SWEATS WAKING YOU	↓ ESTROGEN + SEROTONIN	DYSREG-ULATED HYPOTHALAMUS → HEAT & ADRENALINE	WAKING DRENCHED, SHEETS SOAKED, FEELING DISORIENTED AND ANGRY
RESTLESS LEGS / BODY DISCOMFORT	↓ ESTROGEN + SUBSEQUENT DOPAMINE & IRON ISSUES	SENSORY DYSREGULATION, DIFFICULTY IGNORING BODY SENSATIONS	"ANTS IN YOUR LEGS" OR BODY FEELS ITCHY, FIDGETY, IMPOSSIBLE TO STAY STILL

Neuro-Hormonal Sleep Decoder

HIGHLIGHT OR CIRCLE YOUR SYMPTOMS

↓ = DECLINING, DECREASE IN, LOW ↑ = RISING, INCREASE IN, HIGH

SYMPTOM	HORMONE/ NEURO-TRANSMITTER	WHAT'S GOING ON	WHAT IT FEELS LIKE
CHRONIC PAIN INTERFERING WITH SLEEP	↓ ESTROGEN + SEROTONIN ↑ INFLAMMATION	HEIGHTENED PAIN PERCEPTION, POOR REPAIR AT NIGHT	TOSSING & TURNING TO AVOID PRESSURE POINTS, HIPS OR BACK ACHE, FEELING BETRAYED BY YOUR BODY
FEELING UNREFRESHED DESPITE 7–8 HOURS	↓ ESTROGEN POOR SLEEP ARCHITECTURE (LESS REM/DEEP)	ND BRAINS LESS EFFICIENT AT RESTOR-ATIVE PHASES, SENSORY DISTURBANCES THROUGHOUT	WAKING GROGGY, HEAVY, AND ALREADY NEEDING A NAP
ANXIETY-DRIVEN INSOMNIA (OCD LOOPS)	↓ GABA + SEROTONIN ↑ CORTISOL	OBSESSIVE THOUGHT LOOPS, MENTAL REHEARSALS, CATA-STROPHIC SCENARIOS	LYING AWAKE REVIEWING IMAGINARY DISASTERS & MENTALLY DRAFTING APOLOGY EMAILS
SNORING AND/OR WAKING GASPING FOR AIR (POSSIBLE UNDIAGNOSED SLEEP APNEA: NOT ALL PEOPLE WITH IT SNORE)	↓ DOPAMINE & GABA + TESTOSTERONE, GROWTH ↓ HORMONE & LEPTIN ↑ GLUTAMATE, CORTISOL + NOREPINEPHRINE	REPEATED NIGHTTIME OXYGEN DROPS, TRIGGERING INTENSE "FIGHT-OR-FLIGHT" STRESS RESPONSES THAT DISRUPT ESSENTIAL RESTORATIVE SLEEP	INTENSIFIED EXECUTIVE DYSFUNCTION, SEVERE MEMORY LAPSES, EXTREME EMOTIONAL REACTIVITY, AND PROFOUND BRAIN FOG, OFTEN WORSENING EXISTING ADHD OR AUTISM SYMPTOMS

Reset Your Bedroom: Mini Declutter/Prep Guide

Your sleep environment is not just aesthetics—it's neuroscience. Sensory input, light, clutter, and temperature all directly affect circadian rhythm, cortisol release, and how your ADHD/autistic+ brain processes rest. A few small, evidence-backed tweaks can make your bedroom a true sleep ally.

1. Clear Visual Chaos

• Research shows clutter is linked with higher cortisol levels and lower perceived well-being (Saxbe & Repetti, 2010).

• Keep only what you need in sight—nightstand, bed, one calming object. Store or cover the rest.

• Try a quick 5-minute "sweep" each evening—clothes off chair, clear surfaces.

2. Optimize Sensory Input

• Too many visual stimuli keep your brain "on call." ND brains especially struggle with disengagement.

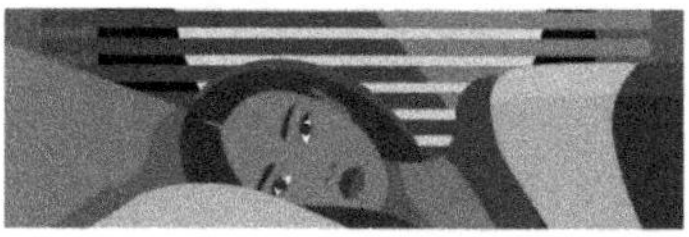

• Soften overhead light; use lamps or red-spectrum bulbs at night.

• Weighted blankets or breathable textiles can reduce physiological arousal and anxiety (Peled et al., 2023).

3. Control Light & Sound

• Blackout curtains or an eye mask support melatonin production by blocking artificial light (Cho et al., 2016).

• White, pink, or brown noise reduces environmental disruptions (Gao et al., 2022).

• Avoid scrolling in bed—the blue light hits your suprachiasmatic nucleus and delays sleep onset.

4. Temperature & Air

• Ideal sleep temp is around **60–67°F (15–19°C)**. Cooler temps trigger the body's natural thermoregulation for sleep onset (Okamoto-Mizuno & Mizuno, 2012).

• Air purifiers can improve perceived sleep quality for those sensitive to allergens or odors.

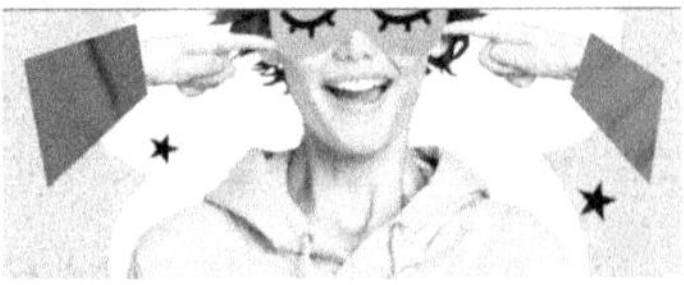

5. Ritualize the Reset

• Pair your reset with an existing nightly habit (ex: brushing teeth).

• Keep it under 10 minutes: light tidy, lights dimmed, sound on, phone out of sight. Consistency trains the brain: this space = sleep.

Wind-Down Rituals Checklist

☑ Warm shower or bath

☑ Make a cup of your favorite sleepy-time chamomile tea if that's your jam. If you've never tried it, go for it. You might love it, and it might actually help you!

☑ Dim lights & screens (I dare you to turn your phone off. And let's next-level it: I double-dog-dare you to put your phone out of your reach.)

☑ Music, white noise, or pink noise

☑ Gentle stretches or yoga (the irony is on not lost on me here, but yes, try yoga!)

☑ Journaling or voice-noting to brain-dump thoughts

☑ Write tomorrow's priority & let it go (I actually text myself my top big priorities for the day, and if I'm feeling extra fun, I'll leave myself a funny, encouraging note like 'GO GET 'EM TIGER!' You'd be surprised at the impact seemingly small gestures like that can have sometimes.)

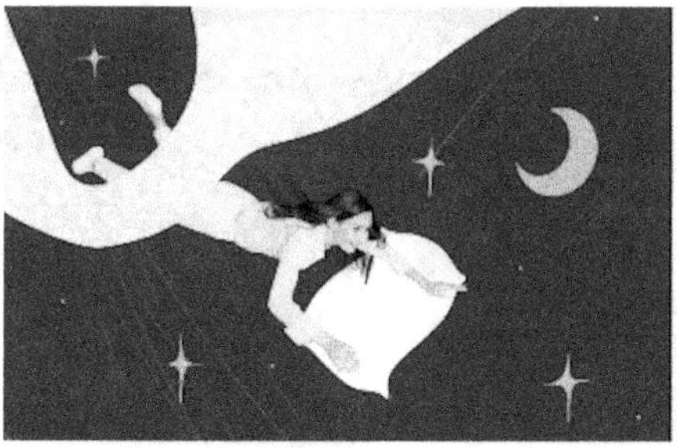

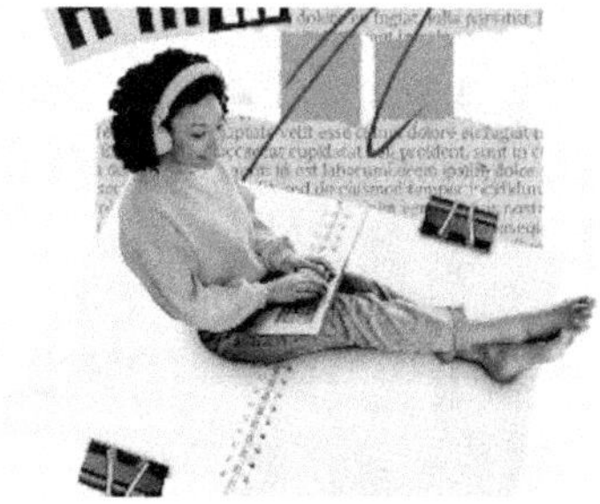

Bonus Tip: Don't Just Lie There

If all else fails and you're still awake — here's something that can actually help, even if it feels backwards: get out of bed.

If you lie awake in bed too long, your brain starts to associate the bed with wakefulness and stress rather than rest. This is called **stimulus control**, and it's one of the most effective behavioral treatments for insomnia.

Instead:

- Move to another room (even just a hallway).
- Keep lights dim.

• Do something quiet & boring (fold towels, read something familiar, sip warm tea).

• Return to bed only when you feel drowsy again.

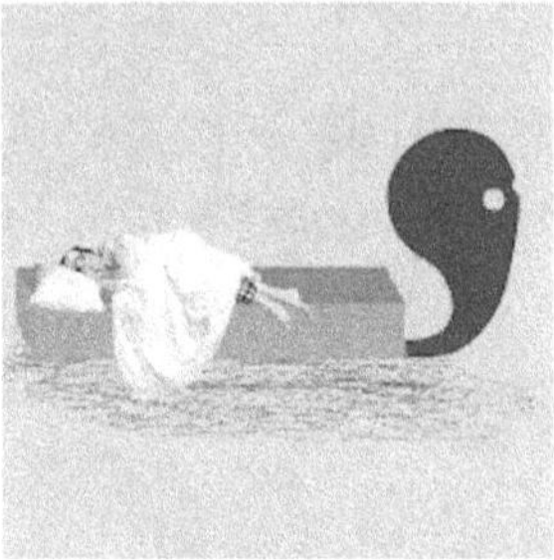

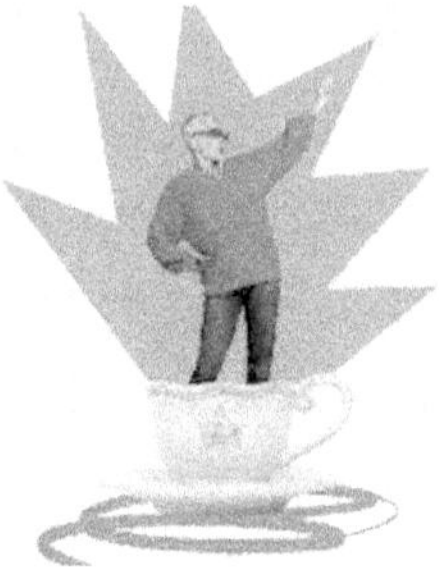

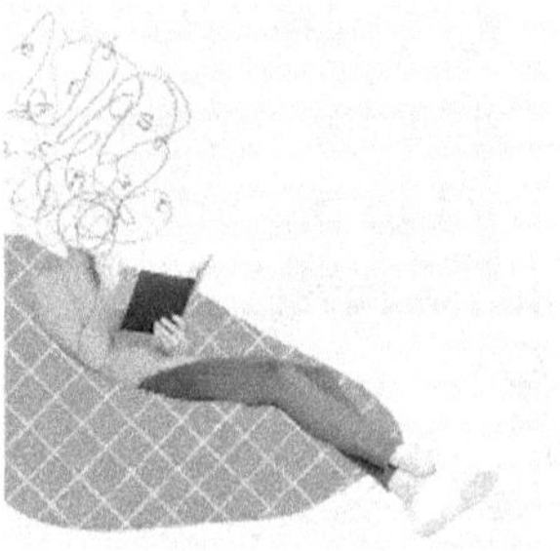

Your bed should be for sleep and intimacy — not existential dread and podcast rabbit holes.

5-Minute Morning Reset

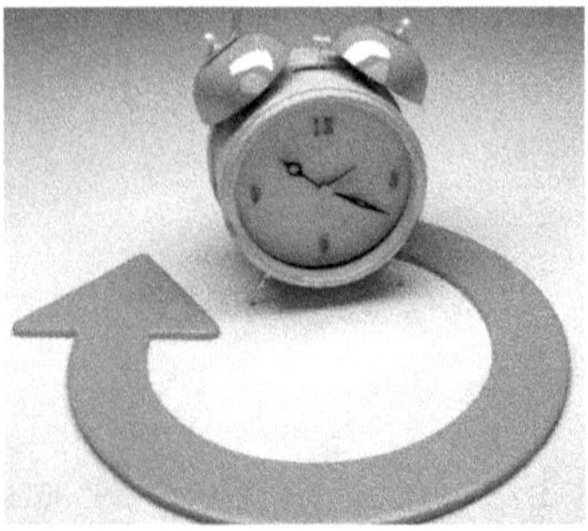

☑ Drink water ☑ Step outside, even briefly

☑ Move your body (stretch, march in place)

☑ Eat something with protein

☑ Say: "I did the best I could."

Print the "What Actually Counts As Rest Mini-Poster" in your Online toolbox. *Be a rebel: print multiple copies and stick them in your office, on the bathroom mirror, in your freakin' car if it helps!*

Emergency Insomnia Cards

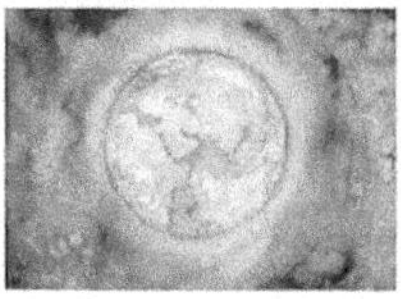

***

Rest

still

counts.

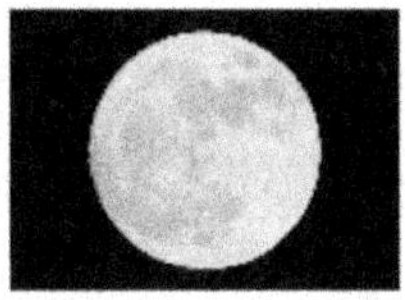

Body scan:

face,
shoulders,
arms,

legs.

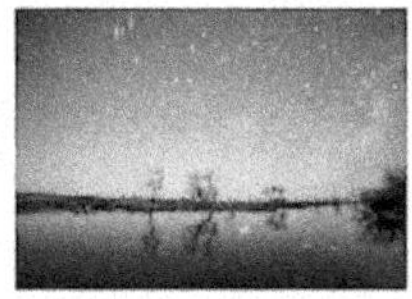

If awake
after 20
minutes,
get up &
do
something
boring.

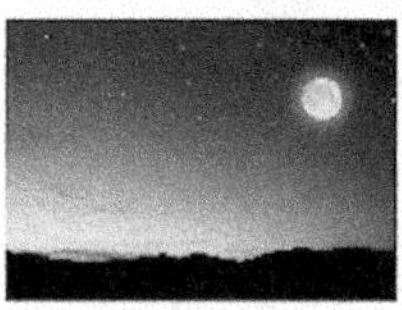

Don't
check your
phone.

It's a liar.

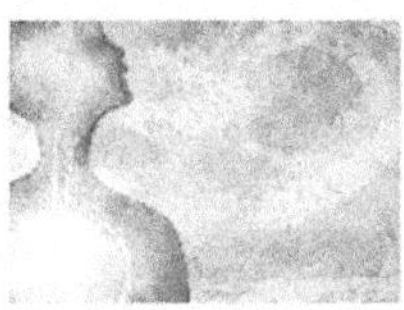

Hands on
belly.
Breathe.
You're
safe.

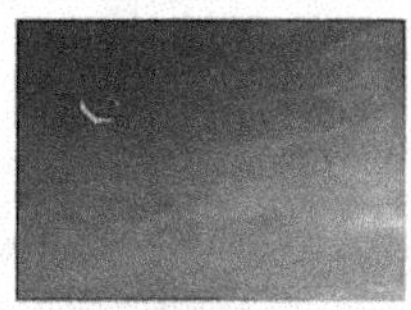

Even just
lying here
is good.
You're not
failing.

Available in your Online toolbox. You know the drill. QR code on p. 24 & p. 38 if you forgot.

A NOTE for PARTNERS

Sleep struggles are one of the most visible symptoms to partners — they see the tossing, turning, and exhaustion.

If you're reading this as a partner/spouse:

✅ Believe them — this is real.

✅ Avoid minimizing ("just relax" does not help).

✅ Help make the bedroom calmer, cooler, and quieter.

✅ Encourage them to rest without guilt — even if it means saying no to plans.

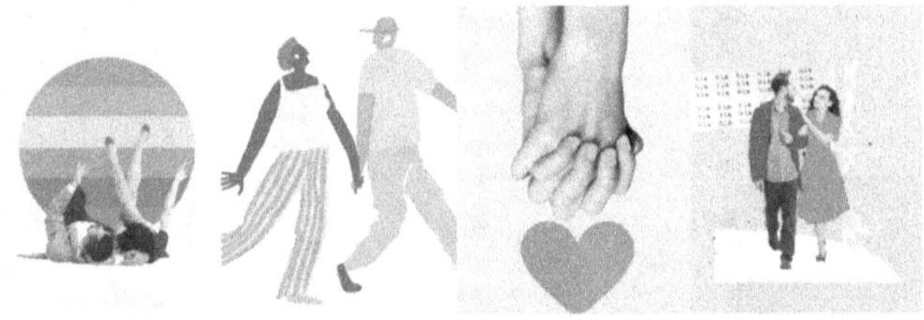

More tools and conversation starters for partners can be found in Chapter 5.

Why "Colored" Noise Can Help Brains Settle and Sleep

Not all "white noise" is the same. Engineers sort steady sounds by how energy is spread across frequencies:

- **White noise**: equal energy at every frequency—like a constant hiss.

- **Pink noise**: energy drops as frequencies rise (a 1/f profile). It sounds softer, less "hissy."

- **Brown (Brownian) noise**: energy falls off even faster ($1/f^2$), so it's deeper—think distant surf.

So why can these help restless, ND brains?

Two big mechanisms show up in recent research:

01 Masking & stability.

A consistent sound floor reduces the salience of unpredictable peaks (doors, trucks, partner snoring) that trigger micro-arousals. A 2022 systematic review of sound interventions during sleep reports that "steady sound can reduce the perceived loudness and intrusiveness of environmental noise" and improve subjective sleep continuity (Gao et al., 2022). In short: fewer "gotchas" for an already hyper-vigilant system.

---

02 Brain-rhythm nudging (entrainment).

Gentle, low-frequency-rich sounds—often delivered as **pink-spectrum** or brief tones timed to your slow waves—can amplify deep sleep oscillations that support memory and recovery. A 2023 meta-analysis concludes that acoustic stimulation "reliably enhances slow-wave activity and boosts memory performance" in adults, when timed to the sleeper's own brain rhythms (Wang et al., 2023). Another clinical review sums it up: acoustic stimulation can "enhance slow oscillations and spindles," key features of restorative sleep architecture (Lustenberger et al., 2022).

"Steady sound can reduce the perceived loudness and intrusiveness of environmental noise." (Gao et al., 2022)

Acoustic stimulation can "enhance slow oscillations and spindles." (Lustenberger et al., 2022)

Which color for whom?

- **White noise** masks best in uniformly noisy spaces but can feel "sharp."

- **Pink noise** is often more comfortable long-term and shows the most evidence in sleep/learning studies.

- **Brown noise** can feel soothing for ND folks who like low-end rumble; evidence is emerging, but user tolerance is high.

How to use it

- Keep it **quiet-to-moderate** (about 40–50 dB bedside). If you need to shout over it, it's too loud.

- Run it **continuously** through the night to prevent arousal from "the noise turning off."

- If you're curious about memory benefits, look for **"pink noise"** or **"deep sleep"** profiles; save closed-loop, EEG-timed stimulation for supervised studies or medical-grade devices.

Great FREE (or free-tier) noise options

- **myNoise** (iOS/Android/Web) – fully tunable generators including pink/brown; strong free tier.

- **White Noise Lite** by TMSOFT (iOS/Android) – lots of loops; free with ads.

- **Atmosphere: Relaxing Sounds** (Android) - customizable mixes; free.

- **Noice** (Android, open source) - simple, free colored-noise generator.

- **Spotify/YouTube** - search "pink noise 8 hours" or "brown noise sleep;" free with ads.

- **Sleep Sounds by Sleep Jar** (Alexa skill) - free voice-activated loops.

For me personally, I have the White Noise Lite app and use the Brown Noise option on my phone when I'm traveling. Occasionally when away from home, I will choose the thunderstorm loop or ocean waves crashing, but at home, I have a small Mooka air purifier in my bedroom that produces white noise at a perfect volume for me. Also, no matter where I am, you can be certain that if there aren't blackout curtains, I will be rigging blankets or whatever I find to block out even the smallest sliver of light coming through a window at night. Complete darkness is non-negotiable for me. Hall light coming through the crack under the bedroom door? Nope. With sound, find what type seems to work best for you and at what volume, and roll with it. You never know what might help regulate your nervous system and block out both physical and mental noise that often contribute to sleep disruption.

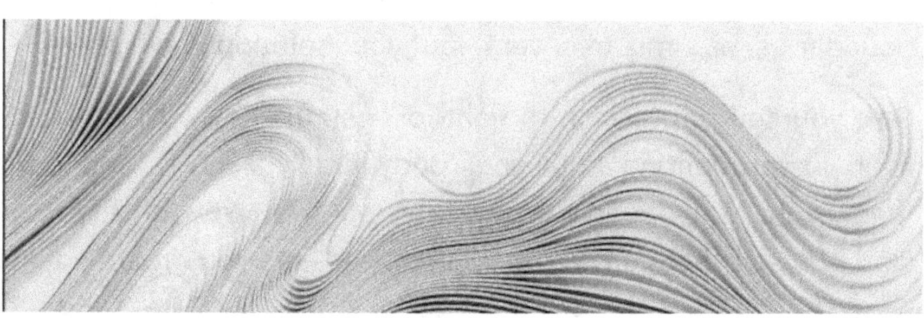

🩶Closing & Encouragement

Here's the thing about sleep: you cannot hack your way around it.

You can fake it for years (decades, if your brain was as stubborn as mine), but eventually your body will start cashing the checks your brain keeps writing. Sleep is not the cherry on top of wellness-it's the fucking foundation. Without it, everything else will collapse.

If your nights are haunted by tornado-brain chaos, intrusive thoughts, and/or hormonal sabotage, hear me: you are not weak, broken, or lazy. You are running a marathon with bricks strapped to your ankles. And no doctor, no wellness influencer, no well-meaning relative gets to tell you that exhaustion is "just in your head." Don't let anyone dismiss your exhaustion. Fight for your sleep like your life depends on it. Because it does.

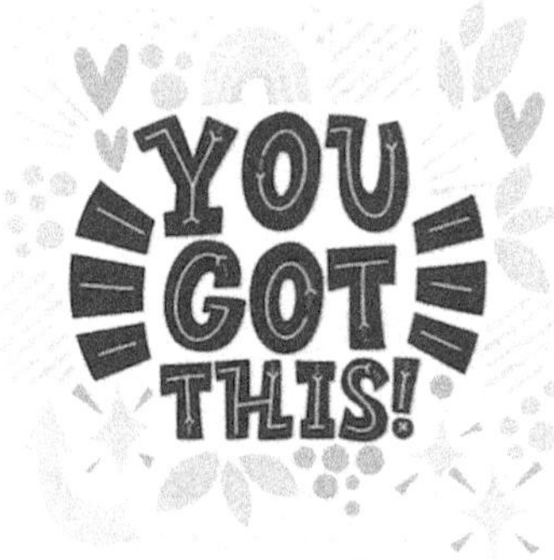

Finding what works may take time, trial and error, and a few spectacular failures (oh, hello, Ambien). But don't give up before you find your version of relief. It might be hormone therapy, a magnesium supplement, ADHD meds, an antidepressant (and yes, maybe even a sleep med for you), therapy, boundaries, or a mix of several-but your solution is out there.

Give yourself permission to fight for rest, to keep advocating, to keep experimenting until your body finally exhales and says: thank you. You deserve more than survival. You deserve the kind of sleep that-forgive the cheesiness-lets you dream again.

Chapter 5

Cultivate Connection Without Masking

Theme: Authentic Belonging

Goal: Rebuild genuine, nourishing relationships—with yourself and others—by dropping the mask, setting honest boundaries, and tackling the real challenges neurodivergent brains and bodies face in midlife with hormonal shifts.

* * *

Neurodivergence and midlife hormonal chaos don't just mess with your brain and body.
They shake up every relationship you have.

For most of us, masking—hiding your ND traits, faking "normal," camouflaging struggles—was a survival tactic. But it also left you feeling disconnected and unseen, even in a room full of people.

Hormones make it harder to "keep up the act," and for

many, the pain of pretending finally outweighs the fear of being "too much."

The truth? You deserve to drop the act, to connect without shrinking yourself, and to build the kind of chosen family where you can actually breathe.

This chapter is about education, communication, and boundary-setting for you and your partner and/or loved ones so you can weather the storm together instead of apart. It's about getting real about sex if that's important to you, authentic intimacy that's right for you, and the ways perimenopause and neurodivergence amplify the disconnects (and how to fix them).

What You'll Find in Chapter 5:

☑ **Unmasking Myths & Truths Mini-Guide** – Reframe old beliefs and see your authentic self as worthy of love and belonging.

☑ **Relationship Inventory Worksheet** – Map who fills you up, who drains you, and where it's safe to drop the mask.

☑ **Expanded ND Social Scripts (cheat sheet)** – Boundary-setting prompts for texts, conversations, and social situations—no apologies, no people-pleasing.

☑ **Rejection Sensitivity Reality Check Reference** – Remind yourself what's ND, what's hormone-fueled, and what's total BS.

☑ **Emergency Exit List** – Pre-approved, no-guilt reasons for bailing on events, people, or plans.

☑ **Partner Connection Section: Sex, Intimacy & Honest Communication** – Everything partners need to know about intimacy with a neurodivergent person experiencing hormonal fluctuations, with research-backed advice and real conversation scripts.

Welcome & Why This Matters

The Stakes Are Higher Than We Think

Divorce rates currently peak in midlife, and new studies suggest that miscommunication about libido changes, pain during sex, and emotional volatility plays a major role (Trujillo, 2026; Yildirim et al., 2023).

Add the complexities of neurodivergence—like rejection sensitivity dysphoria (RSD) and sensory overload—and/or the isolation + lack of resources for gender-diverse folks, and relationships can fracture without support.

Chapter 5 teaches you how to:

✔ Reclaim authentic connection

✔ Find your people

✔ Speak your truth

✔ Refuse to apologize for what makes you real

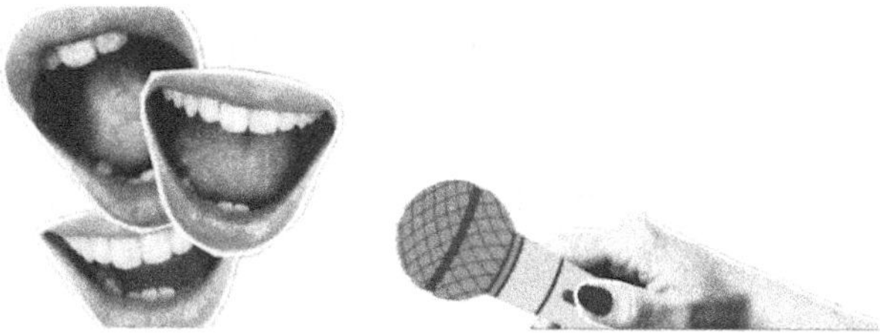

⚡ Quickstart Instructions

1 Read the "Unmasking Myths & Truths" mini-guide to challenge your fears about authenticity.

2 Complete the "Who Gets My Energy?" Relationship Inventory before making new plans or commitments.

3 Try one of the expanded ND Social Scripts next time you need to set a boundary.

4 Print the "Rejection Sensitivity Reality Check" for days you feel like hiding.

5 Use the "Emergency Exit" list for awkward social escapes.

6 Flip to the Partner Connection section—including the new Sex, Intimacy & Communication guide.

7 Remind yourself daily: You're not asking for a favor. You're asking for the care you deserve.

First, a story...

ADHD & Peri/Menopause + Relationships: The Dopamine Tango

The hardest part of being completely unaware that both perimenopause and ADHD were conspiring against me wasn't the disorganization or the missed deadlines — it was the isolation.

I felt utterly alone, and I felt hopeless. Living in a brain that constantly betrayed me and having no words for the crime was inexplicably awful. I watched colleagues seemingly glide through perimenopause like it was nothing.

I felt like I was the only one struggling super hard, and it made me feel like a total loser. **I quit my marriage AND my career in perimenopause, unaware of the hormonal havoc my undiagnosed ADHD and OCD were apparently exacerbating.**

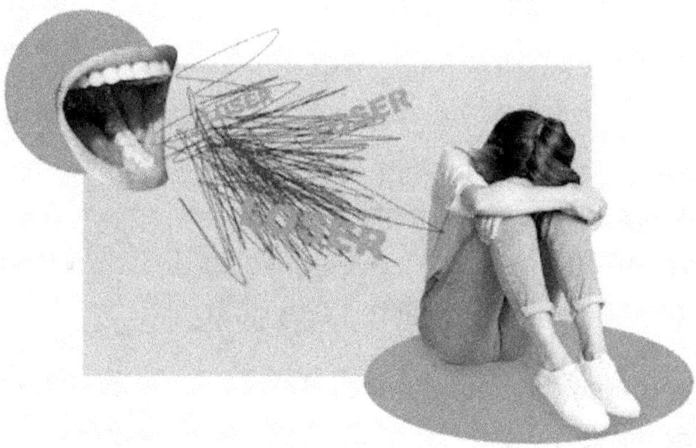

But this part is important: society always wants to frame menopause as a binary gendered issue, and that is wrong.

For one thing, cis women aren't the only people who experience disruptive hormonal fluctuations, midlife or otherwise. To brazenly quote myself in the opening of this book:

> Many trans men, nonbinary people, and other gender-expansive AFAB individuals also live through puberty, menstruation, pregnancy, surgical menopause, perimenopause, and menopause-related hormonal shifts that can affect attention, mood, cognition, and treatment response. (Me, 2026)

People whisper, oh too bad, she lost her job, she got divorced.

Yes, those are sad things. But you know what's sadder and more accurate? My husband lost a wife, and my university, colleagues and students lost an amazing professor. That's the **real** reality.

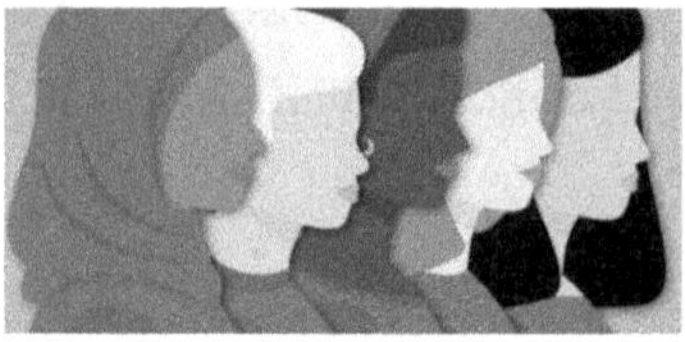

EVERYONE LOSES when people experiencing major hormonal shifts aren't supported.

Undiagnosed ADHD + OCD (amplified by midlife hormones) choreographed most of my relationships, both professional and personal, and not always gracefully. I confused intensity for intimacy, chaos for chemistry, and crisis for connection. I over-gave until I drowned. I apologized until my own name tasted like guilt.

I've only realized recently that I was in a constant state of **limerence** until my relationship with my current partner ...

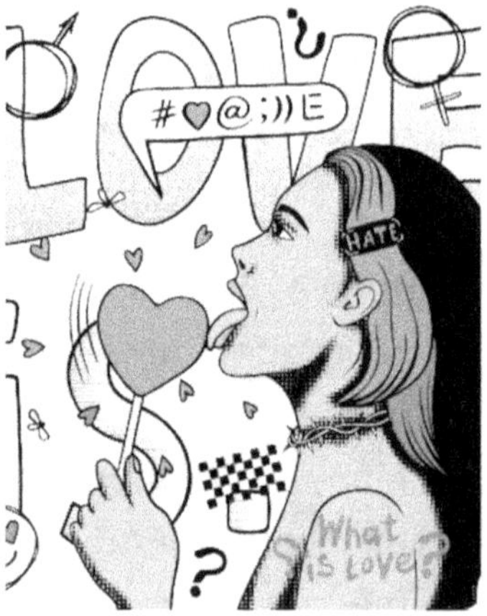

Quick tangent ... for those who know what limerence is, bear with me; but it's important and related if you don't, so allow me to explain, because I only learned of this concept a couple years ago, and examining my life through this new lens with both neurodivergence and peri/menopause has been revelatory.

Limerence is a state of intense, involuntary romantic obsession with someone, characterized by intrusive thoughts, idealization (crystallization), and a deep desire for reciprocation, leading to euphoric highs or despair depending on perceived responses, and it's often one-sided and driven by uncertainty, not necessarily true love.

The concept and term were coined by psychologist Dorothy Tennov in 1979. Basically, it involves an all-consuming focus on someone, with mental energy spent analyzing their actions and longing for them to return the intense feelings.

Some studies present evidence of a consistent correlation between limerence and anxiety, depression, substance use, and anxious attachment style (Willmott & Bentley, 2015).

Limerence has also been linked to trauma, and Willmott and Bentley suggest that childhood abandonment or neglect may correlate with the likelihood of experiencing limerence.

It's also been associated with PTSD as well as OCD, so yeah, my life and relationships framed through this concept have been enlightening.

I "accidentally" married my boyfriend at 21 and stayed for 24 years, ultimately because of people-pleasing and caring what everyone except me thought about it.

OK, it's way more complex than that, and I did say yes. But I was young, and ignorant, and undiagnosed.

I craved connection, and I took a marriage proposal as solid proof someone loved and accepted me.

For a person with low self-esteem, this was a big deal.

We separated multiple times before we even had kids.

And then I did what so many desperate folks do:

I decided that children would fix everything. And so we had two.

I will say, my kids are the biggest blessing of my life.

But having them didn't fix anything. I was always restless. In the end, I know that my ex-husband and I should have never married, or that we should have divorced the first time I wanted to get out. But then, we wouldn't have our kids.

There's no point in regretting this past for me. It brought me to this moment and is part of who I am now, cliché as that sounds.

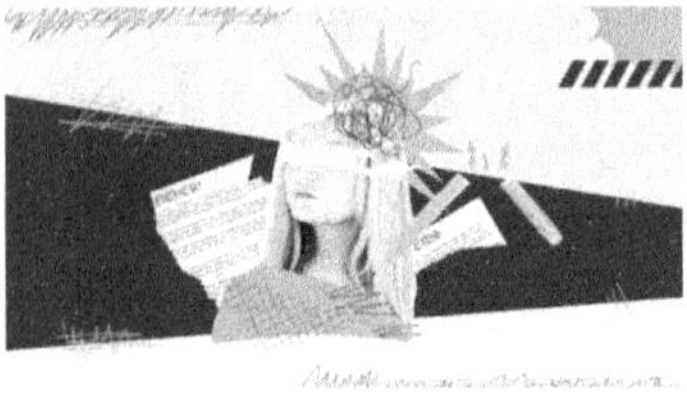

I experienced constant limerence as a teen, I was drawn to people who loved the sparkle but not the mess — the charisma, not the crash. I thought if I could just keep dazzling, no one would notice I was dying inside from the exhaustion of being misunderstood. But I was also drawn to people just like myself at times as well, and so the mutual chaos and crashes became relationships baked in toxicity and iced with excessive unhealthy coping mechanisms.

Now I see the pattern. And yes, it "explains everything." But it doesn't erase responsibility or pain — it just gives it shape. I can look back and say, *"Oh, I wasn't crazy. I was coping."* That's not hindsight; that's liberation. And shedding the shame is the ultimate liberation.

Unfortunately, I was in a relationship that was never meant to be. It was never going to work, no matter how much couples and individual therapy we did (for the record, we did a lot).

Hands down, the hardest thing I've ever done in my entire life was finally getting the courage to put myself first and leave a marriage that was never right for me, fully aware of how much pain my act of self-preservation would inflict on so many people, first and foremost my kids and their dad.

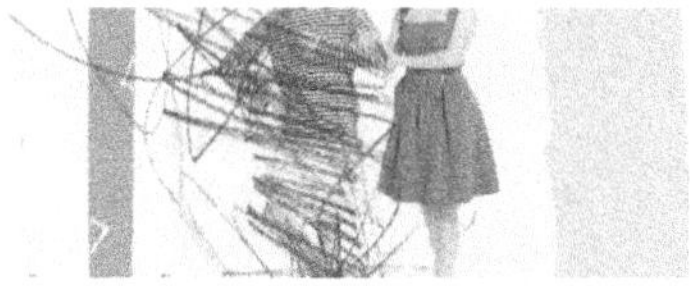

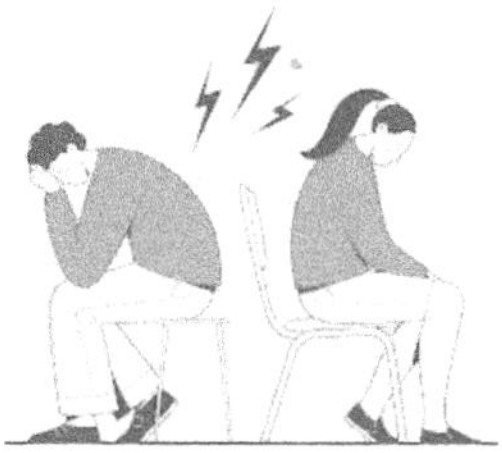

There is no sugarcoating that in any conceivable way. It sucked for everyone. But every relationship is different. And so many can be salvaged with proper support and communication in place. If you're struggling in yours, you are not alone! Healing is possible. There is a light at the end of even the darkest tunnel. Walk towards it. You've got this.

Unmasking Myths & Truths Mini-Guide

MYTH: "If I show the real me, I'll lose everyone."

TRUTH: The ones who matter want the real you. Everyone else is just background noise.

MYTH: "I'm too sensitive/awkward/ emotional/ weird."

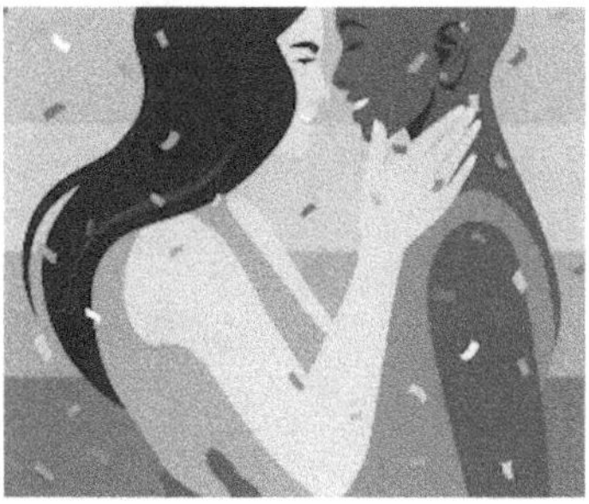

TRUTH: You're perceptive, honest, and more tuned-in than most people can imagine. That's a gift.

MYTH: "Setting boundaries = being rude."

TRUTH: Boundaries are how healthy relationships survive—especially when ND and hormones make your energy precious.

Who Gets My Energy?

RELATIONSHIP INVENTORY WORKSHEET

PRINT AND USE BEFORE EVERY MAJOR PLAN, HOLIDAY, OR SOCIAL EVENT.

NAME / RELATIONSHIP	HOW I FEEL AFTER TIME WITH THEM	DO I MASK? (Y/N)	DO I FEEL SAFE TO UNMASK? (Y/N)	WOULD I CHOOSE THIS IF I HAD NO GUILT?
SARAH	AWESOME	NOPE	HELL YEAH	ABSOLUTELY

Reflect:

-Who truly fills your cup?

-Who drains it?

-Where do you feel most like yourself—and why?

ND Social Scripts (Boundary-Setting Cheat Sheet)

No more asking for permission—just clear, confident self-advocacy.

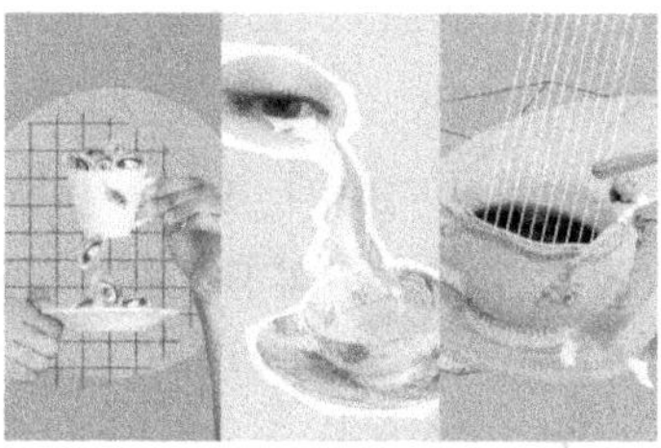

• "I want to see you, but I need to keep it low-key. I may need to leave early, ok?" If you notice me heading out or getting quiet, that's me taking care of myself, not you.

• "My brain's full today, so I'll reply when I can. If you don't hear from me, just know I still care." Some days are just bandwidth management mode—I promise I'm not ghosting, just recharging.

• "I care about you, but I need some solo time right now to reset." Taking a break helps me show up better for both of us later.

• "My social battery's dead—it's not personal. If I duck out early, it's just a reboot, not a rejection." I'll be back when my brain has a fresh charge.

• "Let's do something quieter or with fewer people—my nervous system's on high alert lately." Noise and crowds are tough right now, but I still want to hang with you.

• "Can we reschedule? My hormones are feral, and my brain is in a blender. I'd rather see you when I'm more myself." You'll get a better version of me if I take a raincheck today.

Partner Connection Section:

Intimacy, Sex & Honest Communication: Real Talk for Partners about Hormones

Why This Matters: Massive hormonal fluctuations don't just affect mood and memory—they can absolutely upend sex and intimacy, and these hormonal shifts aren't limited to midlife. They can happen after pregnancy, after an oophorectomy (removing ovaries produces surgical menopause), and taking any type of HRT (MHT, GAHT, birth control) can be a contributing factor as well if levels aren't correct for a person's desired outcomes. Genital dryness and pain (genitourinary syndrome of menopause, or GSM) are *common* but rarely talked about.

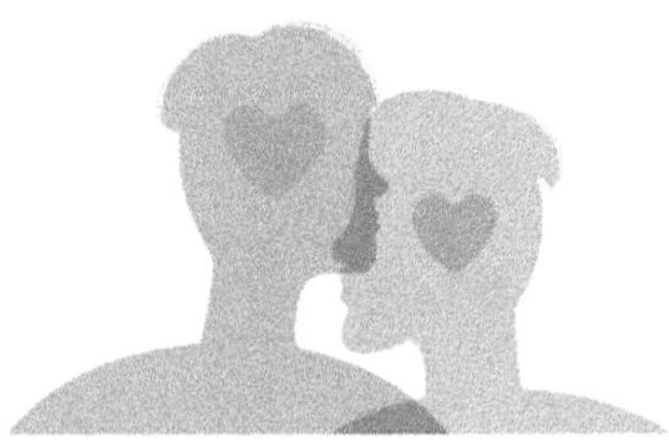

Up to 80% of women experience vaginal dryness [due to estrogen deficiency in tissues], and more than half report painful sex during and after perimenopause [due to the dryness and resulting atrophy] (North American Menopause Society, 2024; Kroese et al., 2024). But it's crucial to stop framing these issues as issues that only cisgender women face.

For neurodivergent people regardless of gender identity, it's amplified:

- Sensory issues make discomfort harder to ignore.
- Shame or communication blocks make it hard to speak up.
- Hormonal changes tank libido and increase sensitivity to rejection.

If you don't talk about it, it breeds resentment and loneliness. This isolation can be exponential for LGBTQIA+ folks, but especially trans and nonbinary people who already face exclusion in clinical settings and research on menopause, and are more likely to be neurodivergent as well.

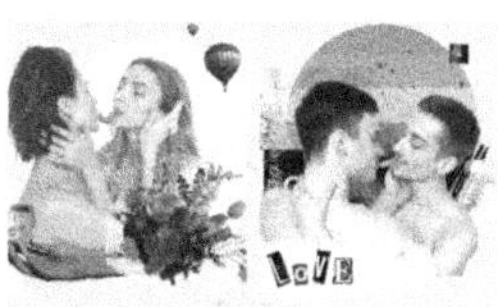

"Current menopause scholarship and health promotion overwhelmingly target cisgender women and rarely consider the complex hormonal pathways through which trans and gender diverse people experience both menstruation (Schwartz et al., 2022; Zwickl et al., 2024) and menopause (Cheung et al., 2023; Mohamed & Hunter, 2019; Sobel et al., 2024; Toze & Westwood, 2025)" (Drysdale, Karasu & Watson, 2026).

This isn't just about sex and it's not just about cisgender heterosexual couples — it's about connection, trust, and keeping relationships alive and thriving for all humans.

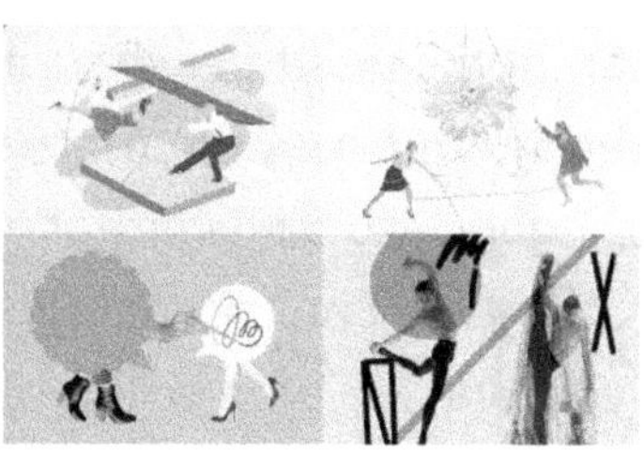

Why This Section Exists: Relationships can become fragmented when big hormonal shifts occur, often due to sexual disconnect, emotional volatility, miscommunication, and unaddressed shame or pain. This is preventable with honesty, mutual learning, and radical empathy. Your relationship can absolutely thrive if both partners face these changes together.

Some Research Perspectives

"Sexual pain and vaginal dryness are the most commonly reported causes of declining sexual activity in midlife. For **neurodivergent [cis] women**, these symptoms are compounded by **sensory processing differences** and greater difficulty accessing appropriate care or self-advocacy" (Kroese et al., 2024).

Furthermore, **trans and gender diverse people** "continue to struggle finding language, clinical guidance, or supportive care environments that acknowledge their experiences. Mainstream menopause resources may compound disparities for trans and gender diverse people through gender-exclusive language, cis-normative imagery, and limited acknowledgement of **diverse hormonal trajectories**" (Drysdale, Karasu & Watson, 2026).

And: "Staying engaged with your pelvic anatomy will keep that anatomy healthier than if you ignore it. Just like the rest of your body, **your pelvic anatomy needs maintenance and attention** [regardless of whether or not sex is a priority for you]. That attention can be purely exercise-focused. Anything that helps you stay in tune with your pelvic floor and genitourinary structures is going to benefit your long-term pelvic wellness" (Firefox Allen, 2026).

What Partners Need to Know

- It's Not About You: Pain and low libido are a physical/neurological issue. Not a referendum on attraction, love, or "failing" as a couple.
- Shame is Real: Many ND brains feel broken, guilty, or avoidant. If they're not initiating, it's not rejection—it's survival.
- Communication Heals: Unspoken resentment breeds distance. Honest, shame-free talk about sex and intimacy is uncomfortable *and* essential.
- Help, Not Pressure: Support means learning, listening, and offering help—not taking it personally or applying pressure.

Intimate Connection Evolves: There are options—lubricants, moisturizers, new routines, non-penetrative intimacy, and medical treatment (local estrogen, etc.) that make sexual pleasure possible again if that's a priority for you. Know that it's ok if it's not.

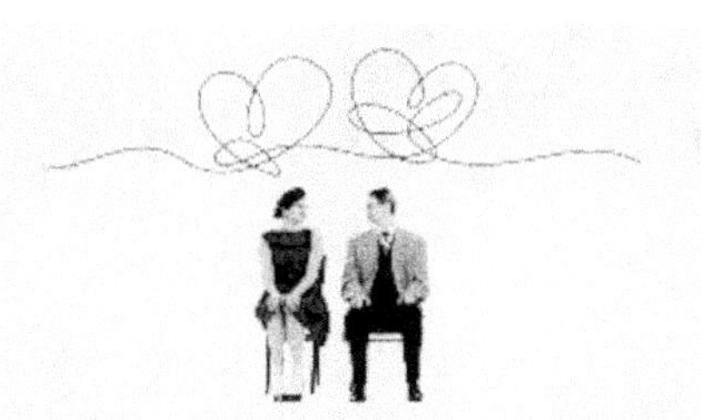

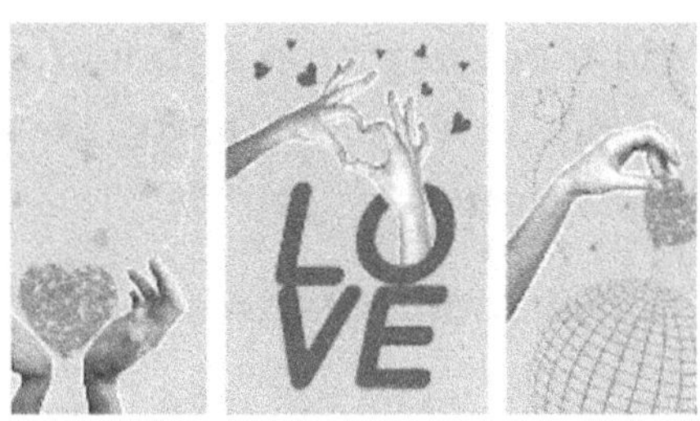

* * *

Script Prompts for Real Conversations

For Those Experiencing the Shifts to Say:

• "I want to be close, but sex feels uncomfortable right now. Can we talk about ways to make it better for both of us?"

• "My body's changed, but it's not about attraction. It's about what I need to feel safe and comfortable."

• "I need patience and understanding. This isn't easy for me to talk about, but I want us to be a team."

For Partners to Ask or Say:

• "What can I do to help you feel more relaxed or safe when we're together?"

• "I read that menopause can cause painful sex and dryness—do you want to talk about what you're going through?"

• "I'm not going anywhere. We'll figure this out together, at your pace."

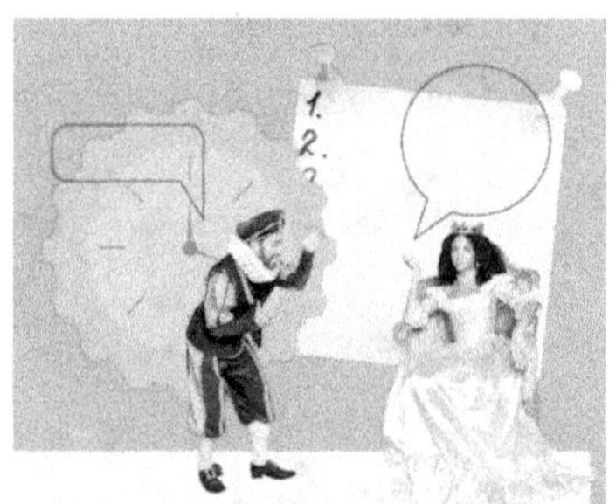

"Is there anything I should stop doing, or try differently, so this feels better for you?"

Conversation Starters:

"What kind of intimacy do you miss, or wish we could have more of—even if it's not sex?"

"Do you want to try new ways of being close, like cuddling, massages, or just hanging out together with no pressure?"

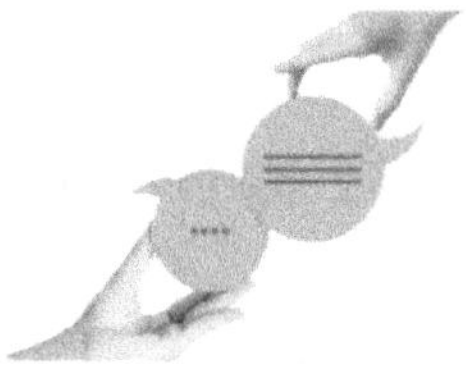

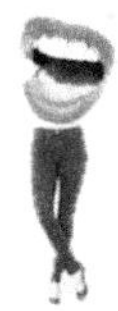

"Would you feel comfortable talking with your doctor or a pelvic floor therapist about this together? I want to support you."

RSD Reality Check

I wish I were taking about Record Store Day here, but alas, no. **RSD (how we lovingly refer to Rejection Sensitivity Dysphoria) isn't a character flaw.**

It's a known neurodivergent brain feature (regardless of it not being a symptom in the DSM-5), amplified by estrogen swings. Most people are too busy with their own shit to plot your social demise. Seriously. You have survived every perceived rejection so far.

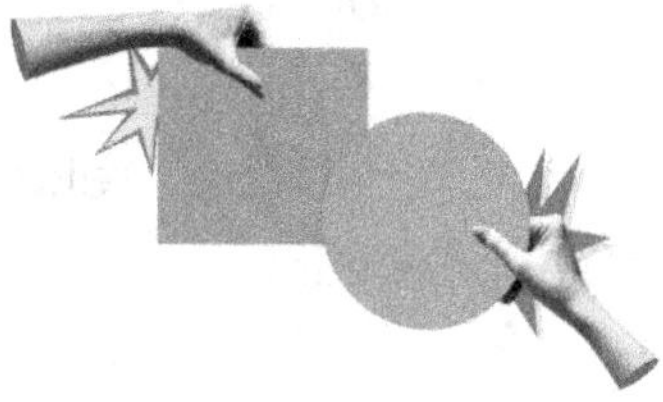

One "no" doesn't erase your worth. Breathe, move, vent, text a friend, or drop a note on the ADHD Peri Punks and/or the NeuroPause Collective Instagram accounts. They get you. They got you.

* * *

🚪 Emergency Exit List

Because not every social situation is survivable—and that's okay.

"I promised myself I'd be home by 9."

"My dog needs me."

"I'm hitting my sensory limit."

"I have an early start tomorrow."

"Thank you for understanding—I need to take care of myself tonight."

The Power of Unmasking: Living Authentically in Midlife

Unmasking, especially during menopause and for the neurodivergent, means letting your true self—brain, body, and needs—show, even when society expects you to hide. Suppressing stims, ignoring discomfort, laughing on cue, and striving to appear "normal" may have once served as self-protection or helped maintain relationships and employment. However, menopause intensifies sensory reactions, emotional swings, and cognitive shifts, making those masks difficult to maintain. **Suppressing your needs starts to drain more energy than it preserves.** Physical and emotional symptoms—like hot flashes, weakened self-filter, or sudden irritability—break through your mask. Meltdowns may now occur in public, not just in private. This isn't a personal failure, but your body and brain refusing to uphold impossible standards as hormonal and neurological changes dismantle the mask you built.

Unmasking isn't about willpower; it's a process riddled with fear and hope. Initial cracks may show up as anxiety—fears of being judged, misunderstood, or "too much"—bred from years of criticism or pressure to conform. The urge to shrink yourself and hide can feel overwhelming. Yet, honesty—admitting you need quiet, soft clothes, or stimming after a draining meeting—can bring a wave of relief. Breathing feels easier. Starting small, with one trusted person or in a safe space, each truthful moment chips away at shame. Even a single conversation about sensory overload, though exposing, can foster empathy. Asking for the lights to be dimmed or music turned down takes courage but opens the door to genuine connection.

Unmasking in daily life is radical self-kindness. Start where it's safest: openly fidgeting with jewelry, rocking in your chair, or letting yourself laugh out loud with supportive people. These aren't mere quirks—they're vital ways your body manages energy and stress. At work, disclosing neurodivergence to a trusted colleague can feel risky, but can also lead to understanding and practical support. Sometimes, wearing comfortable clothing—even if it goes against expectations—becomes an act of quiet rebellion and self-care. As a professor, I mostly wore jeans in an environment where the majority of faculty, administrators, and staff dressed up, and no one ever said a thing. Every time you put your needs first, even nervously, you reinforce your worth. Full openness isn't safe everywhere—discretion is important—but choosing authenticity over masking, even in small ways, helps reclaim your true self.

The health benefits of authenticity are broad and significant. **Chronic masking is associated with anxiety, fatigue, depression, and even physical symptoms.** When you stop pretending and honor your needs—such as taking breaks, seeking work accommodations, or prioritizing sensory-friendly environments—stress diminishes. Your nervous system relaxes, sleep and headaches often improve, and creative energy returns. You stop monitoring every social cue, and relationships become deeper as those close to you see your real self. Friends and partners often respond with empathy once your struggles are visible.

🩶 Wrap-Up & Next Steps

Dropping the mask isn't about being rude or reckless. It's about living with your own bandwidth, your own boundaries, and in your own damn body. Connection is medicine—but so is solitude.

Find your people, take the risk, and when rejection stings? Choose a new Emergency Exit and keep going. You are not too much. You are finally enough.

Chapter 6

Craft Your Ongoing Support System

Theme: Sustainable Self-Compassion

Goal: Equip you with the tools, habits, and mindset to stay resilient, adapt as symptoms change, and keep showing up for your badass self—**without** sliding back into isolation, perfectionism, or medical gaslighting.

* * *

You Were Never Meant to Do This Alone.

It's clear that community buffering—the support and validation from others who "get it"—directly reduces the allostatic load (chronic stress toll) of living with intersecting hormonal and neurodivergent challenges (Kooij et al., 2025; Sood et al., 2019).

What You'll Find in Chapter 6:

☑ **Sustainable Support Squad Worksheet** — Map your real-life and online support network—never wonder "who can I call?" again.

☑ **Non-Negotiable Self-Care Menu** — Build your daily, weekly, and monthly self-care habits—without guilt, shame, or burnout.

☑ **Red Flag Radar Worksheet** — Catch burnout and shutdown signs before they spiral, and create your own action plan for recovery.

☑ **Emergency Resilience Menu** — Keep this for those days you need a permission slip to just survive. Tiny wins count!

☑ **"What to Ask for When You Need Help" Script Prompts** — Scripts and prompts for talking to loved ones, providers, and —most importantly—yourself.

☑ **Community & Resource Guide** — A curated list of online spaces, podcasts, neuroaffirming coaching services, neurodivergent + peri/menopausal content creators and groups where you can connect, vent, and get real support. Stories that mix lived experience + science and humor help you build connection, laugh at the absurd, and remind us that we're not alone.

Welcome & Why This Matters

You didn't come this far just to crash and burn at the finish line.

Peri/menopause and neurodivergence are long games, not short sprints.

Your old support systems (if you had them at all) probably didn't serve you—too rigid, too judgmental, or just missing neurodivergent brain experiences and the realities of hormonal fluctuations entirely. It's time for something new, something that evolves with you, and something you don't have to mask or apologize for.

Chapter 6 helps you:

✔ Connect to resources, relationships, and realistic long-term practices so you're not just surviving, but slowly building a life that feels sustainable and supported.

✔ Build the everyday scaffolding (people, systems, reminders, boundaries) that'll help you actually use what you've learned—especially when the next hormone hurricane or executive dysfunction meltdown hits.

⚡ **Quickstart Instructions**

1 Map out your "Sustainable Support Squad"—who are your go-to people, providers, and safe spaces?

2 Choose your non-negotiable self-care practices, and actually schedule them.

3 Use the "Red Flag Radar" worksheet to spot burnout, self-abandonment, or shame spirals early.

4 Check out the "Emergency Resilience Menu" for instant bounce-back on tough days.

5 Review "What to Ask for When You Need Help" script prompts for your providers, loved ones, and yourself.

6 Join a community—online OR in-person. The *ADHD Peri Punks Podcast* Community on Instagram is FREE. (yes, shameless plug) — There is also a private paid subscription community launching in September 2026 that you can join as well: see The NeuroPause Collective on Instagram for more details.

First, a story...

"How did you survive before you knew?"

A Love Letter to Every Undiagnosed Neurodivergent AFAB Person Trying Not to Fall Apart

Before Diagnosis: The Era of 'What the Hell Is Wrong with Me?'

I get asked this question a lot: how did you do everything you did not knowing you were ADHD/OCD and make it through menopause *unscathed?*

First of all, let's clear something up: I was scathed. Very fucking scathed. I just hid it well. Apparently. I understand that now. Before I knew, I thought the chaos *was me*. I thought I was lazy, flaky, dramatic, inconsistent, impossible to love, impossible to fix. Every planner and productivity system was a new religion I immediately betrayed (hello, Pomodoro Method! I'm looking at you. You're awesome but you're not ADHD-proof!). Every apology was a confession of being too much and never enough at the same time.

I was the class clown because laughter was the only language that made sense. I was the over-achiever—but just with things I loved (ironically, I was not a star student who got all A's)—because perfection was the only acceptable mask. I was the burnout professor because academia loves your brain until it stops performing.

After Diagnosis: Grief, Relief, and the Director's Cut

When I finally got diagnosed at 51, I'm not sure I knew what to expect. It shouldn't have been a shock (both my kids are AuDHD), and yet it was. Plus, I had defied the odds and made it all the way through menopause without knowing! But it definitely explains why perimenopause was *actually harder for me personally as a neurodivergent woman.*

Did I expect fireworks? Who the hell knows, but I think I expected relief. What I got instead was grief. Not the grief you see in movies, but instead, the ugly, inconvenient kind that shows up at 3 a.m. with a highlight reel of every time you called yourself lazy instead of lost. Every time you used ableist tactics against yourself and your own ND kids. Every dream you had but abandoned out of fear and an utter lack of confidence and belief in yourself, and perhaps maybe sometimes, just a simple lack of capacity. Because it's never been an issue of capability.

But then came the relief. Finally.

It was like someone handed me the *director's cut* of my own life. Suddenly, every "bad habit" had context. Every meltdown had a map. I started seeing patterns not as pathology but as narrative. My brain wasn't broken — it was just bootlegged from the factory with the "experimental features" still in beta mode.

Life after diagnosis isn't easier, but it's *truer.* The chaos didn't go away; I just stopped calling it failure. I also found other people like me. And those two things together changed EVERYTHING.

The Repetition, the Retelling, and the Why

So yeah. People ask me these questions again and again.

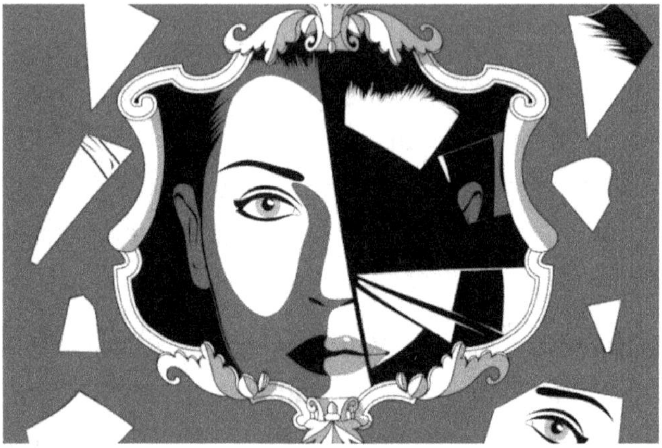

"How did you cope before you knew?" Sometimes I want to say, "Scroll up, I already answered this in April 2024." But every time I answer, someone new exhales for the first time in their life. They join the community I inadvertently created, the one I never realized I needed. And frankly that's incredible.

So I keep talking. I keep writing. I keep dragging my exhausted, sarcastic, subversive, quirky, defiant self back to the keyboard because maybe my survival story is someone else's first step out. Maybe it's a mirror someone desperately needs.

Ultimately, that's reason enough.

* * *

* * *

Sustainable Support Squad Worksheet

FILL THIS OUT. UPDATE AS NEEDED.
YOU DON'T HAVE TO GO IT ALONE—EVEN WHEN YOU WANT TO.

SUPPORT PERSON/ RESOURCE	ROLE (FRIEND, THERAPIST, GROUP)	CONTACT INFO	DO I FEEL SAFE TO UNMASK? (Y/N)	NOTES
SARAH + CHRISSY	ADHD PERI PUNKS PODCAST	INSTAGRAM, FACEBOOK SUBSTACK, TIKTOK, YOUTUBE: @ADHDPERIPUNKS	HELL YEAH	THEY'RE FUCKING HILARIOUS AND REAL.

Non-Negotiable Self-Care Menu

Pick 3 daily, 2 weekly, 1 monthly—post on your fridge, mirror, or lock screen.

• Take a 10-minute walk outside. Yep. Do it. Go. Now.

• Text or call a "safe" friend (ND or otherwise).

• Drink water or herbal tea before coffee (Yes, I know. I know. Many of us ADHDers especially subsist on coffee. But just fucking try this, ok? OK.).

• Write 3 lines in a journal, even if it's just "fuck this. everything sucks. I hate journaling."

• Practice micro-rest: Close your eyes for 60 seconds, or take a power-nap if you can. (I can't. I suck at naps. But if you can manage it, I've heard they're magically restorative. Try it!)

• Do a 5-minute stretch, chair yoga (yes, I said chair yoga), or a gentle dance (Why, yes: I did say gentle dance. So stop your eye-rolling, laughing, or whatever you're doing and start fucking dancing).

• Prep one meal or snack that doesn't make you feel like shit.

• Say "no" once this week and do NOT explain yourself.

• Schedule one "admin" self-care: refill scripts, make an appointment, order groceries, do nothing but breathe.

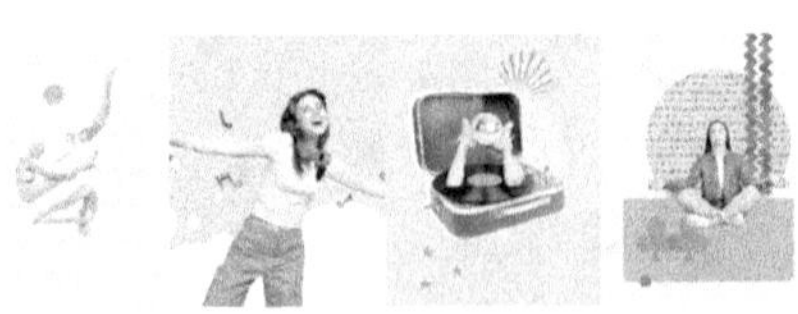

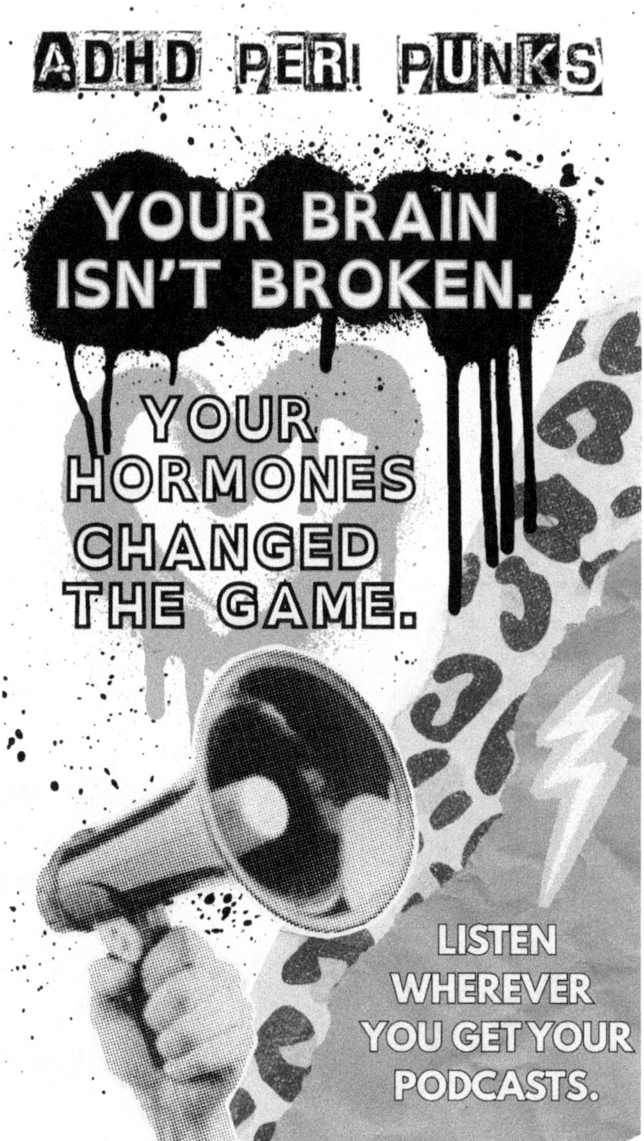

- Listen to an ***ADHD Peri Punks*** episode (or other supportive podcast).

Red Flag Radar Worksheet

REMIND YOURSELF: THESE ARE NOT FAILURES. THESE ARE RED FLAGS, AND YOU'RE A DAMN GOOD DETECTIVE FOR CATCHING THEM EARLY.

EARLY SIGN (BODY/BRAIN)	LAST TIME YOU NOTICED THIS	WHAT HELPED ME RECOVER	WHO CAN YOU TELL / ASK FOR SUPPORT?
TROUBLE SLEEPING			
SNAPPING AT LOVED ONES			
OVERWHELM / SHUTDOWN			
SELF-DOUBT SPIRAL			

Emergency Resilience Menu

You have full permission to:

- Cancel plans. Full stop.
- Eat something comforting, even if it's not "perfect."
- Block, mute, or snooze toxic people online.
- Leave group chats or decline invitations guilt-free.
- Go outside (or just look out a window) and breathe.
- Watch trash TV, rage-clean, cry, or nap.
- DM the ADHD Peri Punks, your therapist, or that one person who "gets it."
- Revisit your affirmation deck or emergency "Validation Playlist."
- Take a shower, or just change your socks. Tiny wins count.

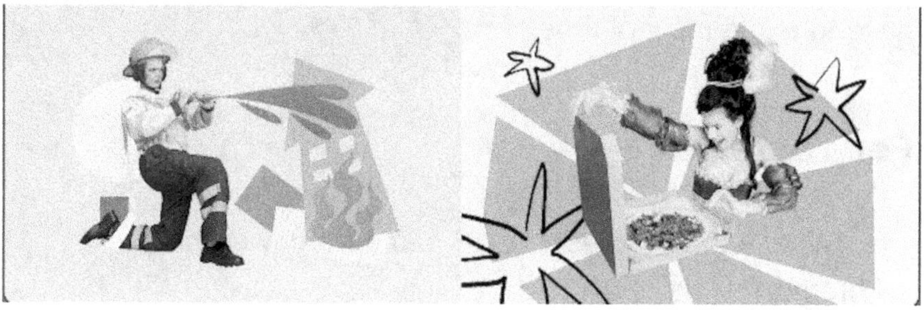

Remind yourself:
Survival is sometimes enough.

What to Ask for When You Need Help (Script Prompts)

For Loved Ones:

• "I need you to just listen, not fix—can you do that for me right now?"

• "Can we problem-solve together when I'm ready, not immediately?"

• "I'm not flaking—I'm protecting my energy. Please be patient with me."

For Medical Providers:

• "I need validation that these symptoms are real, even if you don't have answers."

• "Can we explore options beyond medication—nutrition, therapy, lifestyle?"

• "Please flag my chart for ND and hormonal history so I don't have to explain every time."

For Yourself:

- "What's the smallest thing I can do today to make tomorrow easier?"
- "How would I talk to my best friend if they felt like this?"
- "Which of my affirmations do I need to hear right now?"

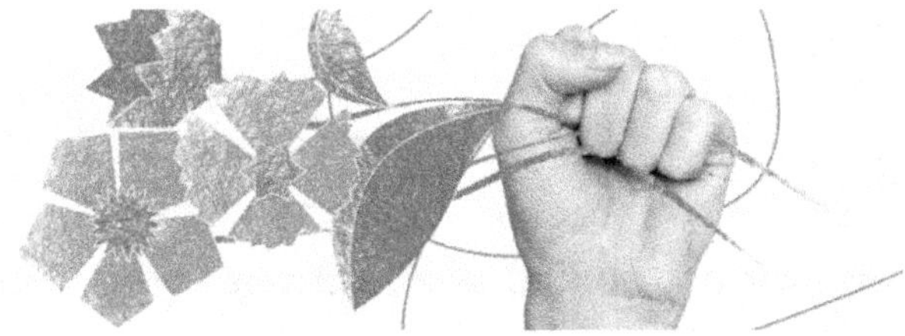

Your Neurodiversity + Peri/Menopause Guide

Finding Your People and Your Professionals

You've decoded the chaos—now, **you need your crew**. This journey is too complex for isolation. The most potent resource isn't a pill or a chart; it's the **radical power of community**, where your "am I the only one?" becomes a resounding "SAME!"

Lived experience is the currency here: **sharing your story** and **hearing others** is how we collectively dismantle the myth that we're something broken that needs to be fixed. But while validation is essential, so is professional, informed support.

The final step is finding your **professional allies**—certified, trauma-informed, and truly **neuro/gender-affirming** coaches and therapists who understand the **intersection of neurodivergence and hormonal shifts** because they are trained in it, and ideally, have navigated it themselves.

No more gaslighting. This resource list is your map to finding both: the healing power of solidarity and the informed guidance of experts.

* * *

Important note on representation

This guide is **not exhaustive**. It intentionally uplifts voices from a **wide range of races, ethnicities, cultural identities, gender identities, sexual orientations, neurotypes, support needs, ages, and nationalities**.

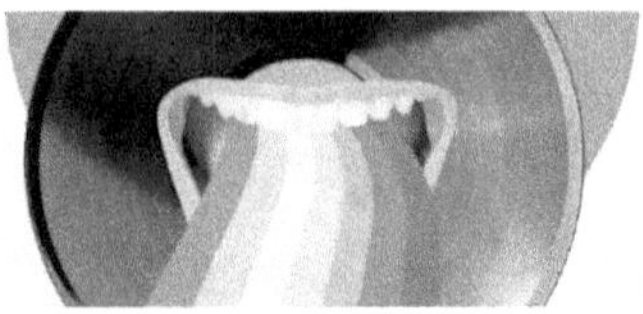

The goal is not completeness, but **connection** — reflecting the many ways people are showing up, sharing knowledge, and building support at the intersections of any neurodevelopmental conditions, perimenopause, menopause, midlife, hormonal fluctuations at any stage of life, disability, identity, and lived experience. Readers are strongly encouraged to keep exploring beyond this list and to seek out voices they don't yet hear often.

☆ **FEATURED RESOURCE** ☆ ***ADHD PERI PUNKS*** ☆

A podcast exploring the intersection of neurodivergence, hormones, identity shifts, rage, systems failure, and survival.

Neurodivergence • Peri/Menopause • Midlife • Gender-Affirming • Anti-Racist • Punk Feminism • Disability Justice • Lived Experience, Evidence-Based & Science-Backed • Diverse Guests • Engaging + Engaged Community • Validation • Anti-Pathologizing

"This podcast exists because too many neurodivergent people are dismissed, misdiagnosed, or gaslit during hormonal transitions. ADHD Peri Punks names what others avoid and does it loudly, honestly, and with heart, humor, and humility."

ADHD Peri Punks Podcast
adhdperipunks.com
@adhdperipunks

Neurodivergence & Peri/Menopause Resource Directory

A Neuroaffirming, Intersectional, Lived-Experience-Informed Guide for Support, Solidarity & Humor

This directory is a living toolkit in and of itself that brings together *clinicians, medical providers, authors, educators, creators, advocates, and community voices* working at the intersection of **neurodivergence, hormones, midlife, relationships, and identity**. Many listed here hold professional credentials *and* lived experience. All perspectives are valid. No pedestal. No gatekeeping.

Please note: Most of the resources in this guide are on multiple social media platforms. I list only the Instagram account for quick reference because this is the platform virtually all are on more than any other. If you aren't on Instagram, you can easily access the other socials + websites for these folks from their IG accounts.

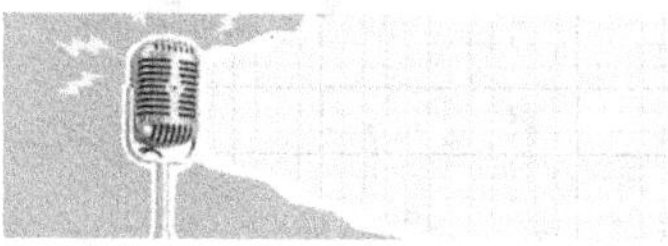

🎙 Podcasts on the Lived Experiences of Intersectional Neurodivergence and/or Menopause

ADHD Peri Punks | Empowering and supporting all people as they navigate the wild expedition of A(u)DHD & peri/menopause. 📍 US / Australia 📲 Instagram: @adhd-peripunks

ADHD AF | Raising hell and ADHD awareness in every country in the world and making sure you know that you are not alone or 'too much,' that RSD is just 'Really Shit Daydreams' and ADHD

IS NOT A TREND. ADHDAF is not a podcast, it's Pirate Radio! 📍 UK →📱 Instagram: @adhdafpodcast

ADHD Women's Wellbeing Podcast | Helping you live alongside your ADHD with more awareness, self-compassion and acceptance. 📍 UK →📱 Instagram: @adhd_womenswellbeing_pod

AuDHD... or just a bit weird...? | Follows host Jon Hill's late-in-life journey through an AuDHD assessment, unpacking lifelong traits, their impact and the coping strategies picked up along the way. 📍 UK →📱 Instagram: @audhdorjustabitweird

AuDHD & me | Unmasked and unfiltered neurodivergent stories, chatting to fellow autistic and ADHD people about their experiences of neurodivergence. 📍 UK →📱 Instagram: @alt_audhd

Black Girl, Brown Girl...Squirrel! A podcast for Neurodivergent Women of Color | For Black, Hispanic, Latina, and Asian women who are Neurodivergent (or wondering if they might be), celebrating the chaos, the brilliance, and the hilarity of brains that don't follow the "default settings." 📍 US →📱 YouTube: @BGBGSquirrel

Black Girl Diagnosed | Amplifying the voices of Black women navigating the intersections of neurodivergence, disability, & mental health. 📍 US →📱 Instagram: @blackgirldiagnosed

Black Girl's Guide to Surviving Menopause | A curated intergenerational exchange, a space for exploration, mentorship, intimacy and vulnerability around life, identity and change. It's the excavation of the things that you need to know, but were never told. It's the guide we wish we all had access to no matter our age. 📍 US →📱 Instagram: @blackgirlsguidetomenopause

Divergent Paths: Neurodivergent Strategies for Late-Diagnosed Adults | Exploring how unspoken expectations, internalized ableism, and cultural myths about productivity keep ND people stuck and what we can do to shift the narrative. 📍 US 📲 Instagram: @drreginaphd

The Genderqueer Menopause Coach | Podcast + Book by Lasara Firefox Allen (mx) about everything genderqueer menopause related, with topics from the spiritual and psychological aspects of menopause to the more physiological and medicalized. 📍 US 📲 Instagram: @genderqueer.menopause

Late Bloomers | The podcast where Rich and Rox Pink—self-proclaimed experts in messing up life—share their raw and unfiltered journey from barely surviving to thriving. 📍 UK 📲 Instagram: @late.bloomers.pod

Late, Not Less | A podcast focused on adulting with ADHD, hosted by Devin Pitts-Rogers on the Attention Different Podcast Network. Designed around radical acceptance, the show destigmatizes ADHD by exploring late diagnoses, rejection-sensitive dysphoria (RSD), and executive function. 📍 US 📲 Instagram: @p0weredbyd0nuts

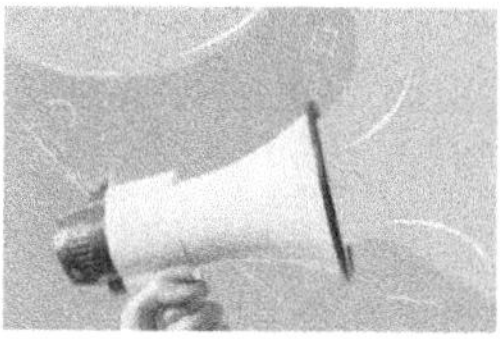

Menopunks | Podcast + Documentary about menopause, perimenopause, quality of life, and the creative process, torching misinformation, setting the record straight about HRT, and giving people the tools to advocate for their bodies, energy, and sanity. 📍 US 📲 Instagram: @menopunks

Mentally A Badass | Keeping it real about mental health, anxiety recovery, and self-growth with raw conversations, expert insights and personal stories. Being vulnerable is badass! 📍 US 📲 Instagram: @mentallyabadass

The ADHD Adults | (In)expertly covers ADHD in adults, sharing evidence-based information and personal experiences. 📍 UK 📲 Instagram @theadhdadults

The ADHD Entrepreneu(her) | For feral AF women in business who refuse to play by the fucking rules. 📍 US 📲 Instagram: @theadhdentrepreneuherpod

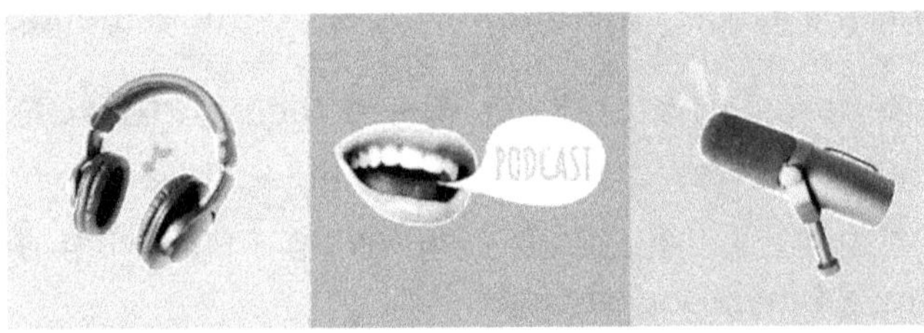

The Dr. Brighton Show | Bringing you groundbreaking research, personal stories, and practical tools to help you confidently navigate your body and hormones. 📍 US 📲 Instagram: @drbrightonshow

This Voice Is Mine | For every neurodivergent mind that was masked, misread, or missed. Where identity is reclaimed & the system gets named. 📍 UK 📲 Instagram: @thisvoiceisminepodcast

TILF (Thoughts I'd Like to Finish) Pod | The group chat where ADHD brains, hot takes, and heart-deep convos collide. Hosted by Dani Donovan, Chris Wang, and Ari Scott, this unfiltered trio says the quiet parts out loud, dives headfirst into the chaos, and somehow makes existential spirals feel like a party. 📍 US 📲 Instagram: @tilfpod

Therapists, Psychologists & Clinicians

Britton, Claire, BOT (she/her) | Occupational Therapist & Founder/Director of Neuroinclusion: Supporting Neurodiversity to Thrive Clinics 📍 Australia 📲 Instagram: @neuroinclusion.au 🧠 Specialty: Neurodivergence Consultations, Therapy & Supports + Developmental & Functional Assessments

Dixon, Mandi L., LPC, NCC (she/her) | ADHD & Menopause Therapist & Coach + EMDR-trained counselor specializing in midlife ND women 📍 US 📲 Instagram: @adhdmenopausetherapist 🧠 Specialty: ADHD, Menopause

Glyde, Tania (they/them/she) | Trauma Informed, Pluralistic, Psychotherapist, Counsellor & Advanced Accredited Gender, Sex and Relationship Diversity Therapist + Researcher, Author & LGBTQIA+ Activist. 📍 UK 📲 Instagram: @queermenopause 🧠 Specialty: GSRD + work with queer, LGBTQIA+, consensually non-monogamous/ polyamorous folks, kinky/BDSM identified, and sex workers

Kahn, Gilly, Ph.D. (she/her) | Psychologist & ADHD Specialist + Author of *Allow Me to Interrupt*; Writer, Clinician, and parent with lived experience 📍 US 📲 Instagram: @drgillykahn 🧠 Specialty: ADHD, Emotional Regulation

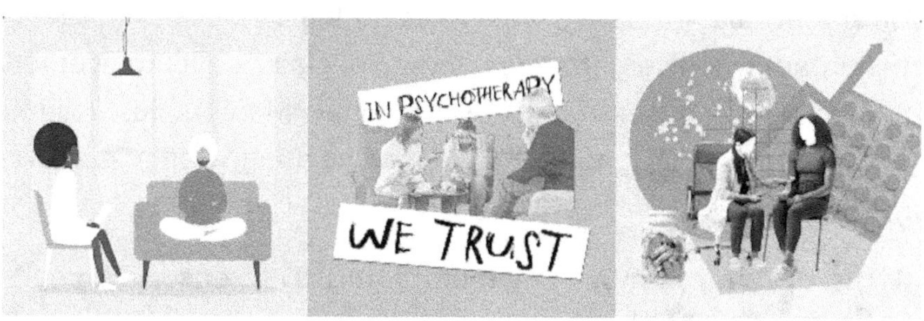

Koliha, Kristin, LICSW (she/her) | ADHD Therapist & Coach: Adult ADHD support with a relational approach 📍 US 📲 Instagram: @welcomehomeadhd 🧠 Specialty: Adult ADHD

McCarty, Calial, M.A., LMHC, CAS (she/they) | Neuroaffirming Therapist & Author of *Naturally Divergent* 📍 US 📲 Instagram: @naturally_divergent_therapist 🧠 Specialty: Autism, ADHD, Assessment.

Moore-Clarke, Shenikka, MSW, LICSW (she/her) | Holistic & Liberation Therapist 📍 US 📲 Instagram: @the.healingvibe 🧠 Specialty: Somatics, Parts Work & Trauma Healing

Murillas, Julie, M.S., LPC, ADHD-CCSP (she/her) | Therapy that gets midlife women 📍 US 📲 Instagram: @juliethep-eritherapist 🧠 Specialty: Peri/Menopause, Anxiety, ADHD & Burnout

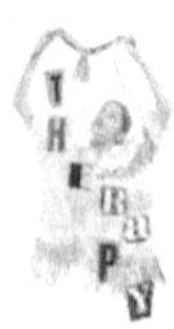

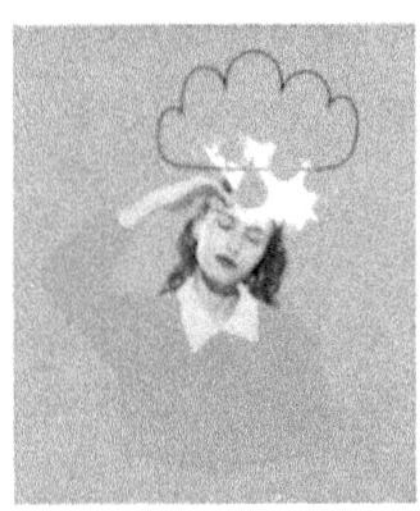

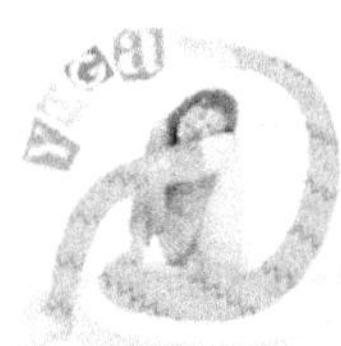

Offord, Emma, Ph.D. (she/her) | Founder & Clinical Supervisor, Divergent Life + Host of This Voice Is Mine Podcast 📍 UK 📲 Instagram: @divergentlives 🧠 Specialty: Neurodivergent Screening & Assessment, Professional Mentorship, Trauma Assessment & Diagnosis, Therapy, Coaching, Somatic Movement & Yoga

Richard, Dylan, Ph.D. (they/them) | AuDHD Licensed Psychologist + Founder of The Punk Psychologist: Queer Psychology with a punk attitude 📍 US 📲 Instagram: @thepunkpsychologist 🧠 Specialty: Trauma & PTSD, Personality Disorders, Sexuality, Queer and Trans Affirming Therapy, Autism, ADHD + AuDHD, Kink/BDSM relationships, Polyamory, Sex Work

Roberts, Lauren, LPC, ADHD-CCSP (she/her) | Relatable Misfit Therapist 📍 US 📲 Instagram: @copinginchaos 🧠 Specialty: ADHD, Anxiety & Co-dependency

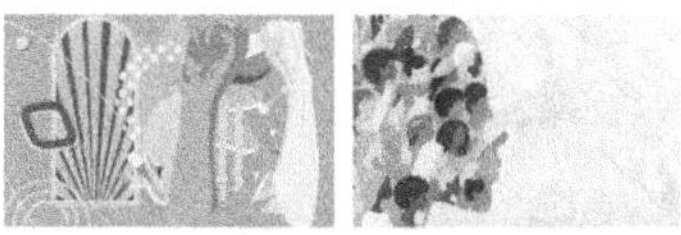

Slonena, Liz, Psy.D. (she/her) | Psychologist & ADHD Coach + Creator of Mindful Hypnosis™ 📍 US 📲 Instagram: @dr.lizlistens 🧠 Specialty: ADHD, Anxiety, Hypnosis

Taylor, Melissa, MSW (she/her) | Clinical Director & Therapist, Ancestral Memory Therapy + CPT, Mindfulness, EMDR, Narrative Therapy & Sensorimotor Psychotherapy certifications 📍 Canada 📲 Instagram: @ancestralmemorytherapy 🧠 Specialty: Trauma & Nervous System Work grounded in anti-racism, anti-oppression & Black feminism

Teumer, Amy, LMHC-QS, PMH-C, ADHD-CCSP (she/her) | Neuroaffirming Therapist 📍 US 📲 Instagram: @amyteumer 🧠 Specialty: ADHD, Autism, and Neurodivergence Evaluation

Tuckman, Ari, Psy.D., MBA (he/him) | Psychologist, Author of *The ADHD Productivity Manual* + four other books on Adult ADHD, International Presenter & ADHD Thought Leader + International ADHD Conference Organizing Committee Chair 📍 US 📲 Instagram: @arituckmanpsyd 🧠 Specialty: Teens + Adults with ADHD, Couples & Sex Therapy

. . .

Wolkin, Jennifer, MFA, Ph.D. (she/her) | Neurodivergent Neuropsychologist, Health Psychologist, Speaker, Poet, ADHD Thought Leader & Author of *Quick Calm,* Neuroscience and nervous system education made practical, human, and compassionate. 📍 US 📲 Instagram: @drjenwolkin | @adhd_with_drjen 🧠 Specialty: ADHD, OCD, Trauma, Mindfulness, Hormones

Coaches, Educators & Strategists

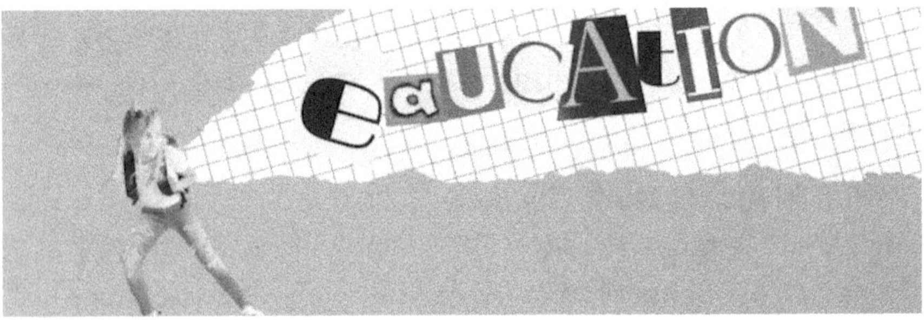

Brockerville, Ellen, B.Ed., B.SpEd., M.Ed. (she/her) | ADHD Educator + Late-diagnosed ADHD Mom 📍 Canada 📲 Instagram: @ellenbrockerville

Cairns, Anj (she/her) | ADHD Coach, Trainer & Speaker training and mentoring ADHD coaches globally 📍 UK 📲 Instagram: @adhdingwithanj

Carder, Meredith, BS-Psych, MBA (she/her) | ADHD Coach & Author + ADDCA-trained coach; midlife ADHD advocacy 📍 US 📲 Instagram: @hummingbird_adhd

Clarke-Boyle, Linzi (she/her) | Therapeutic & Menopause Coach helping women navigate midlife with ease & confidence 📍 UK 📲 Instagram: @linzialignedmidlifecoach

Fregau, Jami (she/her) | ADHD Life Strategies & Education, Nurse + Host of The Neurodivergent Nurse podcast 📍 US 📲 Instagram: @theneurodivergentnurse

Gray, Sera, LCSW (she/her) | ADHD & Perimenopause Therapist & Coach, Wild Lotus Coaching; late-diagnosed AuDHD 📍 US 📲 Instagram: @wildlotuscoachingwithsera

Haynes, Trina (she/her) | ADHD Coach focusing on burnout recovery & capacity-based support at Shimmer 📍 US 📲 Instagram: @myladyadhd

Hirst, Paula (she/her) | Certified Coach for ADHD Women | Burnout recovery & meditation 📍 British in UAE 📲 Instagram: @adhd_and_alchemy

Hopson, Temica (she/her) | Neurodivergent Health Coach Burnout recovery & sustainable wellness 📍 US 📲 Instagram: @tbhwellnesscoaching

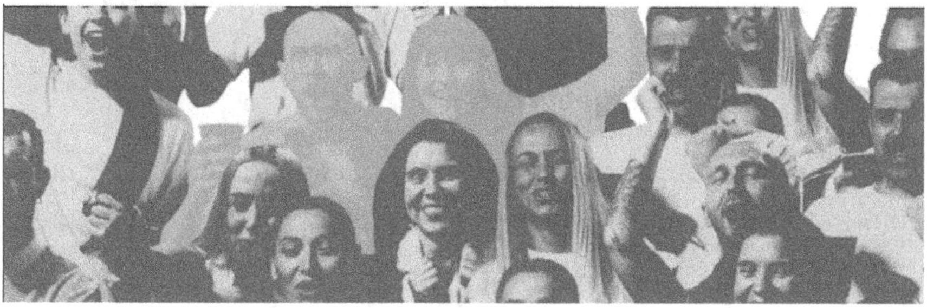

Kamoshita, Kate, MA | ADHD Educator, Poet + Mom 📍 American in Japan 📲 Instagram @learning.compass

Korylak, Beau | Creator of Neurofriendly + Chaos Coach empowering people and families navigating ADHD & Autism 📍 Canada 📲 Instagram: @beaukorylak

Lemansky, Karrie (she/her) | ADHD Business Strategist Host of *The ADHD Entrepreneu(her)* Podcast 📍 US 📲 Instagram: @karrieoutloud

Lawoyin, Asiatu (they/them) | BLACK, disabled, Queer, AuDHD+, atheist, disruptor, SOCIOLOGIST & commUNiTY Coach 📍 US 📲 Instagram: @asiatu.coach

Moryoussef, Kate (she/her) | Late-diagnosed neurodivergent Author, Coach + Host of the ADHD Women's Wellbeing Podcast 📍 UK 📲 Instagram: @kate_moryoussef

Nungaray, Feli, LMFT (she/her) | Neurodivergent Psychotherapist, Coach, and Consultant + Founder of NeuroSeeds Coaching & Consulting 📍 US 📲 Instagram: @neuroseeds_byfeli

Otsuka, Tracy, J.D. (she/her) | Author, Podcast Host, Certified ADHD Coach and Lawyer, ADHD for Smart Ass Women 📍 US 📲 Instagram: @tracyotsuka

Potts, Chelsia, Ed.D. (she/her) | Neurodivergent Educator & Coach, Late-diagnosed; parenting & identity work 📍 US 📲 Instagram: @thedivergenthood

Robertshaw, Suzanne (she/her) | Certified ADHD trauma-informed coach and dyslexia specialist 📍 UK 📲 Instagram: @teachingwithadifference

Scott, Ari | ADHD Business Builder on a mission to help build 100,000 ADHD-owned businesses 📍 🌎 📲 Instagram: @the_adhd_entrepreneur

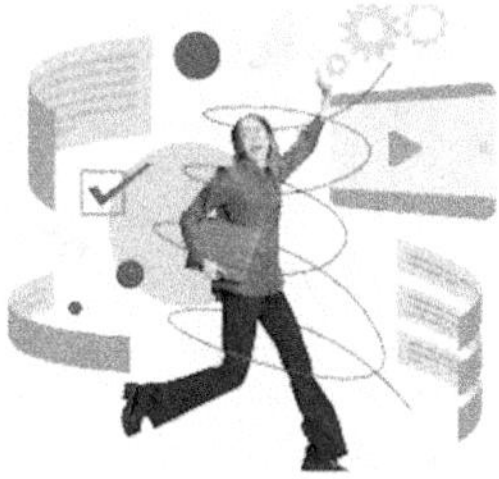 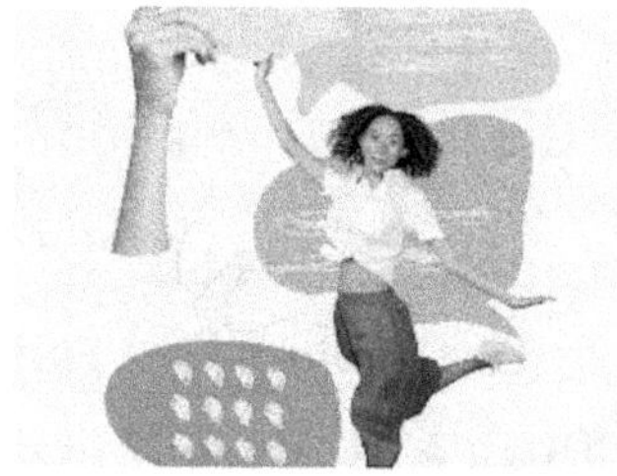

Medical Professionals who Specialize in Hormones, Menopause & Midlife Health

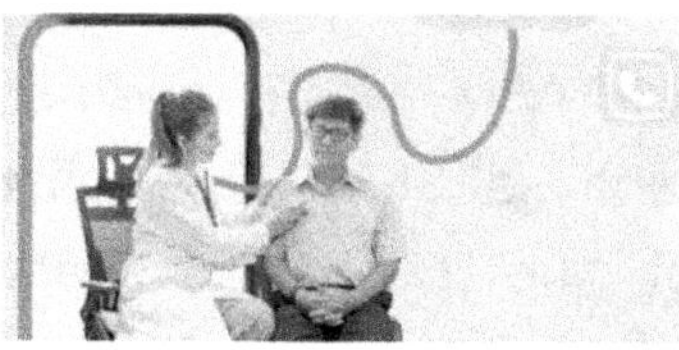

Afsari, Mary Fariba, DO, MS (she/her) | Board-certified OB/Gyn, Author of *Labor: One Woman's Work* & Founder of Fem Forward Health, a full-service mobile healthcare practice providing convenient and compassionate gynecologic and early pregnancy care in communities with long waitlists or limited access to the specialized care they deserve. 📍 US →📱 Instagram: @maryfaribapdx

Andreys, Montserrat, DC, MS, CCSP (she/they/ella) | Sports Chiropractor & Founder of Hey Doc Clinic; Centering the health-care needs of Queer, Trans + BIPOC folx 📍 US →📱 Instagram: @doctor.montserrat

Arif, Nighat, MBBS (she/her) | Women's Health Physician & Author | Menopause education & public health advocacy 📍 UK →📱 Instagram: @drnighatarif

Benkley, Marie, N.D., MCSP (she/her) | Peri/menopause-focused Naturopathic Doctor; Natural and conventional treatment option integration with the most evidence-based care, informed by the best research available + clinical expertise 📍 US 📲 Instagram: @drmariebenkley

Brighton, Jolene, N.M.D. (she/her) | Doctor, Author, Speaker, Podcaster: Board Certified Naturopathic Endocrinologist, Nutrition Scientist, and Clinical Sex Counselor 📍 US 📲 Instagram: @drjolenebrighten

Casperson, Kelly, M.D. | Doctor, Author, Speaker, Podcaster: Board Certified Urologist, Sex Expert &. Menopause Educator 📍 US 📲 Instagram: @kellycaspersonmd

Matsumura, Andrea, M.D. MS, FACP, FAASM, MSCP (she/her) | Sleep Medicine Physician + Menopause Sleep Specialist, Speaker, Consultant & Founder of the D.R.E.A.M. Sleep Method™ 📍 US 📲 Instagram: @drandreamatsumura

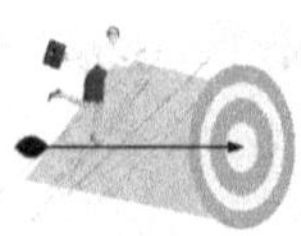

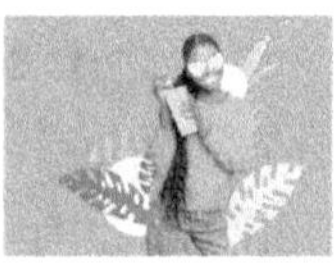

Montville, Michelle, M.D., FACOG, MSCP, DABOM | OB/GYN & Telehealth (Menopause & Weight Care) + Clinical Director-Alloy Women's Health 📍 US 📲 Instagram: @drmmontville

O'Sullivan, Aoife, M.D., MSCP | Physician + Menopause Society Certified Clinician 📍 Irish in the US 📲 Instagram: @portlandmenopausedoc

Phipps, Claire, BSc, MBBS, MRCGP (she/her) | GP & British Menopause Society Accredited Specialist + Advisory Council Member & Menopause Trainer 📍 UK 📲 Instagram: @themenopausegp

Taylor, Barbara, M.D. | OB/GYN & Surgeon turned Menopause Educator + Author: Expert science-based education for all women 📍 US 📲 Instagram: @menopausetaylor

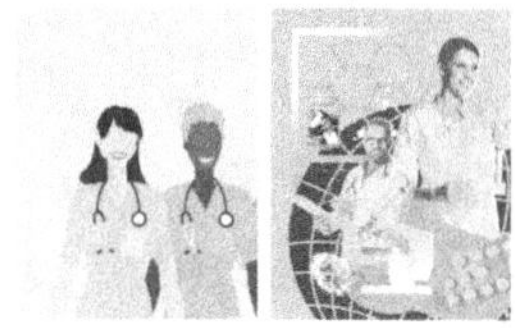

Wall, Helen, MBBS (she/her) | NHS Menopause Clinic GP, Public Health Leader + Media Contributor bridging the gap between professional healthcare and accessible advice for the public Women's health, neurodivergence & menopause + public education UK Instagram: @doctorhelenwall

Weiland, Vanessa, NP, HT, MSCP (she/her) | Nurse Practitioner + Founder of Phases Clinic, Inclusive Menopause & Hypermobility Care US Instagram: @bendymenopause

Community, Identity, Education, Activism & Lived Experience

Allen, April (she/her) | AuDHD Mother, Speaker & Human Design Mentor advocating through visibility. US Instagram: @april_lynn_allen

Burney-Scott, Omisade (she/her) | Founder of the Black Girl's Guide to Surviving Menopause: Charting a path away from the narrow, cis-heteronormative, and predominantly non-Global Majority framing of menopause—what we call the menopause landscape—toward the vast possibilities of the Menopausal Multiverse. US Instagram: @omisadeburneyscott

Canuck, Jennifer (she/her) | Pro-Age Diva + Silver GenX-er aging fiercely and fabulously. Canada Instagram: @the_silver_canuck

Comeau, Ronide (she/her) | Artist & Mental Health Fairy Godmother + Illustrated advocacy & emotional literacy US Instagram: @kikoteroro

Corinna, Heather (they/them) | Queer Feminist Activist, Author, Educator, Artist, Teacher, Organizer & Innovator + Founder, Director, Designer & Editor of Scartleteen (Queer Sex Ed For All) 📍 US ➔📱 Instagram: @heather.corinna + @scartleteenorg

Davis, Ayanna Sanaa (she/her) | Award-winning Autistic Artist + Podcast Host, Autism Advocate & Author 📍 US ➔📱 Instagram: @phenominallyautistic

Deaf Queer Resource Center | National Deaf QTPOC LGBTQ-led 501(c)(3) nonprofit organization 📍 US ➔📱 Instagram: @deafqueer

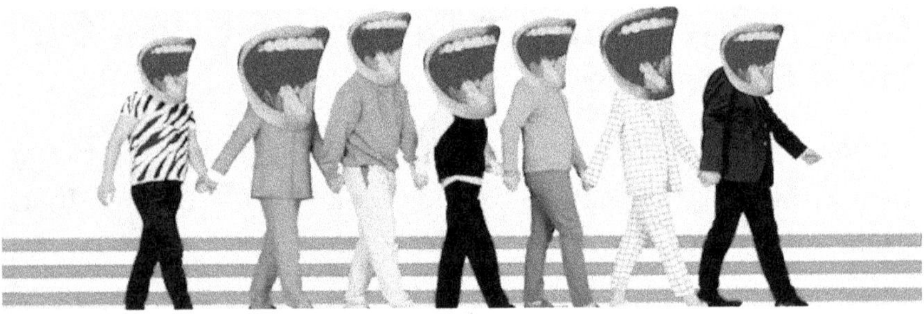

Devereaux, Savant De'Shawn (he/him) | AuDHD Artist & Educator + Lived-experience-based advocacy 📍 US ➔📱 Instagram: @savanttheeprodigy

Eltahawy, Mona (she/her) | Founder + Editor in Chief of FEMINIST GIANT & Editor of *Bloody Hell: Adventures in Menopause from Around the World* ➔📱 Instagram: @monaeltahawy

Firefox Allen, Lasara, MSW (they/them/mx) | Genderqueer Menopause Coach & Author | Training providers in gender-affirming menopause care + Support for genderqueer/trans folks 📍 US ➔📱 Instagram: @lasara_firefox_allen

Fung, Erin (she/her) | AuDHD mum of 3 AuDHD kids + Host of the AuDHD & me Podcast UK Instagram @alt_audhd

Hédi (they/them) | AuDHD, queer, demisexual aromantic lived experience Germany Instagram: @autistic_enby_elder

Hill, Jon (they/them) | Podcast Host & Creator of *AuDHD... or just a bit weird...?* UK Instagram: @audhdorjustabitweird

Holmström, Elin (she/her) | ADHD & Autism Educator & Advocate Sweden Instagram: @beesandroutines

Ingram, Chrissy (she/her) | Punk-Informed Neurodiversity Activist & Punk T-Shirt Designer + Co-host of *ADHD Peri Punks Podcast* Australia Instagram: @redpunksocial

International Dyslexia Association | Nonprofit organization dedicated to helping individuals with dyslexia US Instagram: @dyslexiaida

Kaligirwa (they/she/he) | AuDHD (moderate needs), Agender, Creative + Academic | Advocacy, Critique & Evidence Canada Instagram: @blackspectrumscholar

Keaton, Louise (she/her) | Neurodivergent Content Creator, Slow Living & Self-Love US Instagram: @louaffirms

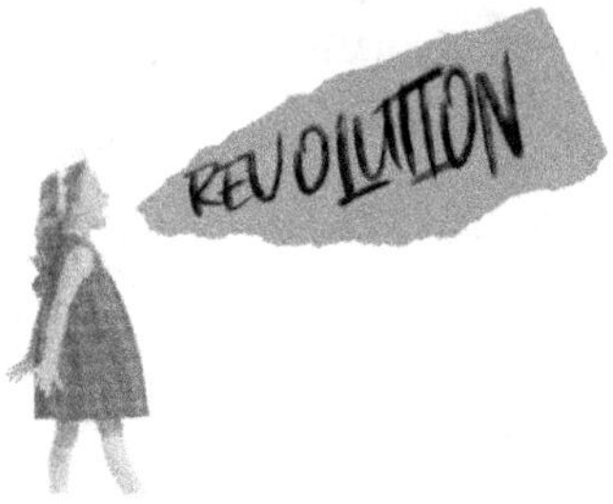

Mears-Reynolds, Laura (she/her) | ADHD Activist, Advocate + Host of *ADHD AF Podcast* & Founder of ADHD AF+ Charity UK Instagram: @adhdafpodcast

• • •

Meyers, Kerise | AuDHD Entrepreneur, Home-Ed SEN Mum, Speaker & Founder/CEO of Inclusion Support Hub, a directory of inclusive services in the UK 📍 UK 📲 Instagram: @mrs.k.meyers

Nichelle, Brittney-Elizabeth (she/her) | Neurodivergent Creator of Practical magic & self-regulation tools 📍 US 📲 Instagram: @brittney.elizabeth

Pharms-Barr, Gabrielle Nicole (she/her) | AuDHD Writer, Brand Strategist & Storyteller, Culture-led Narratives & Brand Identity 📍 US 📲 Instagram: @gabbynikki

R., Alexandra (she/her) | OCD/Anxiety Therapist in Training + Anxious Latina student professional helping you understand OCD, Anxiety & ADHD with compassion and evidence. 📍 US 📲 Instagram: @alexandraisobsessed

Rachel (she/her/xe/xem) | Neurodivergent Content Creator, Graphic Designer + Neurodiversity Educator & Activist 📍 Singapore 📲 Instagram: @autisticasfxxk

Rastrick, Paula (she/her) | AuDHD Patient Advocate, Survivor + Speaker & Hormonal Sensitivity Educator 📍 UK 📲 Instagram: @paula_rastrick

Rosier, Louise (she/her) | Rare Eye Cancer Survivor & Blogger sharing stories of ADHD, Mindfulness, Meditation, Anxiety + Perimenopause 📍 UK 📲 Instagram: @peri_adhd_lulu

Sanders, Melani (she/her) | Perimenopause Educator + Founder of the *We Do Not Care Movement™* 📍 US 📲 Instagram: @justbeingmelani

Shivaramakrishnan, Shruti (she/her) | Illustrator, Creator, Invisible Illness Advocate, navigating life with chronic pain and complex trauma 📍 US ➜📱 Instagram: @chronicallymeh

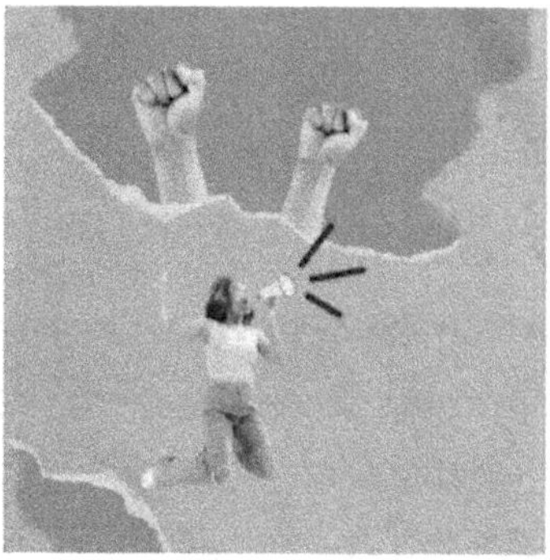

Stevens, Bethany (she/her) | Disabled Sociologist & Culture Critic 📍 US ➜📱 Instagram: @disabethany

Wang, Christal (she/her) | ADHD Coaching CEO + Founder of Shimmer ADHD Coaching 📍 US ➜📱 Instagram: @adhd.christal

Partners, Relationships & Family Support

Borneman, Leann, Ph.D., LCSW, CST (she/her) | Psychotherapist & Coach, Neurodivergent Clinical Sexologist + ADHD Relationship & Intimacy Researcher 📍 US ➜📱 Instagram: @drb_unfiltered

Brown, James, Ph.D. & Brown, Samantha (he/she) | ADHD Coaches & Educators + Hosts of *The ADHD Adults Podcast* 📍 UK ➜📱 Instagram: @adhdadult_james | @mrsaudhd

Davis, Brooke (she/her) | Hormone Science Educator Research-based guidance on midlife relationships 📍 US ➜📱 Instagram: @marriageinperimenopause

Farrise, Kaela, LMFT, LPCC (she/her) | Therapist, Consultant, Researcher + Speaker, MAs in Clinical & Counseling Psychology | Boundaries, Trauma, Mental Health & Relationships 📍 US ➜📱 Instagram: @therapywhileblack

Holderness, Kim & Penn (she/he) | ADHD & Menopause Advocates, Humor-based education on family & midlife 📍 US ➜📱 Instagram: @theholdernessfamily

Iantaffi, Alex, Ph.D., LMFP (they/he) | Author, Sex & Relationship Therapist, Speaker & Host of the Gender Stories Podcast | Healing Justice, Sexual Wellness & Social Justice 📍 US 📲 Instagram: @xtaffi

Rich & Rox (he/she) | Lived Experience ADHD and Autism Authors & Advocates, Creators of the Dubbii Body Doubling App + Hosts of *The Late Bloomers Podcast* 📍 UK 📲 Instagram: @adhd_love_

Robertson, Jesse (he/him) | Menopause Education for Partners Helping spouses understand menopause 📍 US 📲 Instagram: @husbands4menopause

Lifestyle, Diet, Fitness & Nutrition

Clover, Amy, NBC-HWC (she/her) | Neuroaffirming Health Coach Founder of Strong Inside Out; Somatics, Intuitive eating, HAES-aligned, recovery-friendly 📍 US 📲 Instagram: @stronginsideout

Farhat, Ali, B.S. Kinesiology, CMP (he/him) | Certified Menopause Practitioner, Hormone & Metabolic Specialist + Menopause weight & hormone education 📍 US 📲 Instagram: @thatmenopauseguy

Jones, Jerlyn, MS, MPA, RDN, LD, CLT | Media Dietician & Speaker + Gut & Hormone Expert @nutrition4midlife 📍 US 📲 Instagram: @thelifestyledietician_

Miller, Marianne, Ph.D., LMFT (she/her) | Eating Disorder Therapist specializing in ARFID + Binge Eating 📍 US 📲 Instagram: @drmariannemiller

Reid, Diana, MPH, RDN (she/her) | Neurodivergent Nutritionist, Gut Health Expert & Certified Intuitive Eating® Counselor/Coach 📍 American in Luxembourg 📲 Instagram: @theglobalrd

Spence, Shana Minei, MS, RDN, CDN (she/her) | Registered Dietitian, Nutritionist + Author of *Live Nourished* / Non Diet Weight Inclusive 📍 US 📲 Instagram: @thenutritiontea

How to Build Your Own Community—Facilitating Peer Support Spaces

Creating a neurodivergent menopause peer support space may seem daunting, but it's both achievable and rewarding. **You don't have to wait for the perfect group; you can shape one to fit your own values and needs.** Start by choosing a format that fits your comfort level and accessibility—Facebook groups allow for privacy and events, Discord offers real-time moderation and topic channels, while in-person meetings in libraries or community centers suit those who prefer face-to-face connections. Many groups begin with just a couple of people and grow through word of mouth or online cross-posting.

Set clear intentions early with a charter or mission statement that defines the group's purpose and boundaries. For example: "This space is for neurodivergent adults navigating perimenopause and menopause. We honor all gender identities, encourage judgment-free self-expression, and protect privacy." Clarify that participation is voluntary, no medical advice is given, and that lived experience is valued alongside research. Explicitly state your group's commitment to anti-racism, gender inclusion, and neuroaffirming language, with members agreeing to mutual respect. This guidance helps people understand what to expect—and what isn't acceptable.

Effective moderation requires clear rules and consistent enforcement. Set guidelines for confidentiality, respectful disagreement, and boundaries (e.g., "No sharing screenshots" and "No pressure to disclose diagnoses"). Address conflict early: moderators should check in privately when issues arise, remind participants of group values, and, if needed, connect them to outside support. Remove disruptive members promptly to maintain safety and trust. Invite member feedback on rules or formats, and rotate moderator roles to prevent burnout and incorporate fresh perspectives.

Accessibility and intersectionality must be core priorities.

- Start each meeting or chat by inviting pronoun sharing (if members are willing).
- Provide transcripts or captions for virtual gatherings to accommodate varied language processing needs and hearing abilities.
- Continually assess whether your group is welcoming to people of color, LGBTQ+ individuals, disabled people, and those from diverse socioeconomic backgrounds. Partnering with local LGBTQ+ and BIPOC groups can broaden your group's reach and root it in community advocacy.
- Circulate a list of local resources—ND-affirming clinics, menopause-friendly therapists, food banks, etc.—to address multiple member needs.

Facilitators should remain open to ongoing change. Running these spaces brings challenges: maintaining momentum during low-energy periods, managing complex personalities or technical problems, and keeping hope alive during difficult times. **Yet the benefits are clear—members advocate for each other, share practical tips, and offer solidarity through tough nights.** No formal training or large following is needed; empathy, clarity, and willingness to learn together are enough.

Envision the type of space you wish you had found—one where silence and speech are both respected, where whole identities are honored, and no one must choose between important parts of themselves. Your efforts—crafting a mission statement, posting a welcome message, moderating with care—can provide critical support and visibility for people who've long felt unseen.

To begin:

- Draft your group's mission and rules before inviting others.
- Choose a platform that fits your and your community's needs.
- Post conduct and privacy guidelines from the outset.
- Regularly seek feedback, encourage members to suggest topics or formats, and connect with partners who can help expand the group's reach or resources.
- Stay flexible so the group can evolve as new members join and needs change.

Building a community is both radical and practical for neurodivergent people facing menopause. It shifts the narrative from isolation to collective empowerment and wisdom. Facilitators do more than offer connection—they create opportunities for both personal and systemic transformation.

Navigating Nonbinary and Trans Experiences of Menopause

The menopause conversation often assumes a narrow audience —cisgender women, usually white, and not typically those who identify as neurodivergent. This exclusion leaves nonbinary and trans neurodivergent people with a sense of erasure, sometimes outright hostility. You may have faced clinics and resources that misgender you, or felt invisible when group discussions defaulted to "ladies" or "moms." Perhaps you've had to weigh the risk of correcting someone's assumptions against your need for care or community.

Even support groups focused on neurodivergence can slip into gendered language, making you feel like an afterthought. This invisibility is not just an oversight—it's a barrier to health, safety, and belonging. Many gender-diverse people delay or avoid care and community because they expect to be misgendered or dismissed. In these moments, the exhaustion is real—and so is the risk to your well-being.

You have a right to community and care that respect your whole self. *If a community refuses to honor your name and/or pronouns, document the experience and seek another if possible.*

If you're an ally, partner, clinician, or facilitator, your words and actions have a direct impact on whether gender-diverse members feel safe and seen.

- Use people's correct pronouns—make it a habit to ask

for them at every meeting or intake, then actually use them.

- Avoid defaulting to "ladies" or "women's issues" language in materials or events. Say "everyone experiencing menopause," not "all women." When someone corrects you or shares discomfort about language, listen without defensiveness.
- Challenge assumptions in your circles: if a group member jokes about "real women's problems," redirect the conversation and clarify your group's commitment to inclusion.

If you lead a support group:

- Include pronoun introductions, and post guidelines upfront about gender diversity.

Actionable steps help create safer spaces for all.

If you're organizing an event or clinic:

- Ensure forms allow for names and pronouns beyond the binary. Offer gender-neutral restrooms and private spaces for medical discussions.
- Partner with LGBTQ+ organizations to review policies and content for inclusivity gaps.

In Online groups:

- Establish moderation policies that ban misgendering and address microaggressions promptly—members should know your values before they ever have to defend themselves.

The courage required to navigate menopause as a nonbinary or trans neurodivergent person is immense. Every time you advocate for yourself in a pharmacy or challenge exclusion in a group chat, you make the path easier for those who come after. Every time an ally speaks up, another person feels seen instead of erased. Visibility is not about demanding special treatment—it's about affirming that every experience of menopause is valid and worthy of respect, care, and community.

🩶 Wrap-Up & Next Steps

You have built a toolkit, a battle plan, and a support system to survive (and thrive) in the wild intersection of neurodivergence and menopause. You've learned that you're not broken—you're just living in a world that's not built for your wiring. The journey continues, and you never have to do it alone again.

Keep your squad close, your boundaries clear, and your humor sharp.

One last thing: Check out The Neuropause Collective on Instagram @neuropausecollective—where the revolution is just getting started.

Conclusion

This is just the beginning

You now hold a guide that hopefully centers at least part of your experience. Every page has been built to replace confusion with clarity, isolation with community, and shame with pride in your own adaptation.

The chapters of this book are not abstract concepts. They are scaffolding for daily survival and growth.

First, you learned to **Decode & Validate Your Experience in chapter 1**—to see patterns where others saw only chaos, to trust your lived reality even when professionals dismissed you. The symptom mapping gives you tools to track and communicate your symptoms, letting you name what is happening rather than being swept away by it.

Chapter 2: Self-Advocacy Simplified offered scripts and strategies to help you navigate appointments and systemic barriers, so that you are no longer voiceless in the doctor's office or overwhelmed by bureaucracy.

Through **Chapter 3: Executive Function Rescue**, you found ways to adapt routines and break the cycle of self-blame. It also equipped you with concrete techniques to handle sensory overload. You learned how to build sanctuaries, embrace stimming, and give yourself the grace to pause.

Chapter 4 on **sleep**, though, might be the most important one. If you don't have sleep, you have nothing. It is the foundation, so use all the tools in that chapter over and over again, and keep talking to your partner (if you have one) about this.

Chapter 5 provided **relationship communication scripts, empathy exercises, and boundary-setting tools**, so you can connect with loved ones and repair after conflict, while **chapter 6** helped you think more intentionally about the people you surround yourself with and the **importance of community**.

I designed all the tools in this book to help you get on a path to "radical" self-care and a badass mindset. Self-care should not be inherently radical, but unfortunately in the world we live in, it can be a foreign concept pitted against the daily grind of hustle culture, and it is SO much more than bubble baths and retail therapy.

When it comes down to it, these chapters are more than survival manuals. They are blueprints for rewriting the narrative around intersectional neurodivergent peri/menopause. The most transformative lesson, for me, is that **self-knowledge and self-compassion are not luxuries**. They are necessary. You now have practical ways to decode symptoms, advocate for your needs, manage daily tasks, regulate emotions and sensory input, communicate honestly, and foster a mindset that celebrates adaptation over perfection.

Hear this clearly: **You are not the problem.** The systems that overlook, dismiss, or pathologize your experience are the problem. This book is rooted in inclusivity. I wrote it for neurodivergent women, yes—but also for nonbinary, trans, gay, gender-diverse, PGM, and multiply marginalized readers. Too often, health and self-help books erase these voices. In these pages, your experiences are central, not a footnote. Intersectionality is important, and community is essential.

That said, if you take one thing with you, let it be this: you are not alone, and you never have to be again. The curated resource guide is here to help you start to find your people. When we come together—whether online, in person, or simply by reading each other's words—shame melts away. Solidarity grows. Change becomes possible.

Self-advocacy and self-compassion are not acts of selfishness. They are acts of survival and resistance. Use the scripts, checklists, and trackers. Let yourself rest. Set boundaries, even if it feels strange at first. **Redefine what success means for you, not by anyone else's standards.** There is no gold medal for suffering in silence. There is courage in asking for help and wisdom in knowing when to say no.

Finally, I encourage you to think beyond your own odyssey. Share your story, however you are able. Join a support group, or start one if your community still needs it. Challenge clinics, workplaces, and families to do better. Mentor someone who is just beginning to question why everything feels so hard. **Each time you speak up, you make it easier for the next person. Each time you advocate, you chip away at systems built for someone else.** This is how revolutions begin—not with a single voice, but with many, rising together.

If you have made it this far, you are already part of something bigger. Carry these tools with you. Pass them on. Remember: your experience is real. Your needs are legitimate. Your story is valuable—not despite your differences, but because of them.

Together, we are forging a new path for neurodivergent menopause. The map is still being drawn, but it is brighter and broader because you are here. Let's keep building it—one act of courage, one moment of rest, one honest conversation at a time.

Learning to release perfectionism, honor your limits, and recognize the fierce creativity and the resilience you should not have had to have had but that has inevitably carried you this far ... well, those are no small feats.

You are such a badass. You know that, right?

START HERE

Wait, what?

Start here? But this is the end.

Yes, I know. I created this damn thing, which means that I also know you.

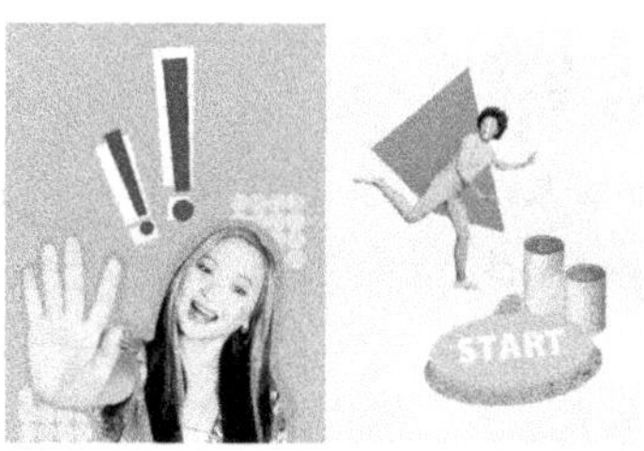

I know you're overwhelmed.

I know that if you're like me, you sometimes just flip to the end of the book, just to see what's going on.

I know that even though I already told you how to use this book at the very beginning, you have probably already forgotten LOL or maybe you skipped that part.

So all of this bears repeating. I GOT YOU!

* * *

One more reminder about your Online Toolbox of printables. All the charts, provider scripts, sample planner layout, affirmation cards, emergency exit and insomnia cards, yeah, all that shit, in a folder for you to print or forget about for 3 years. Either way, it'll be waiting.

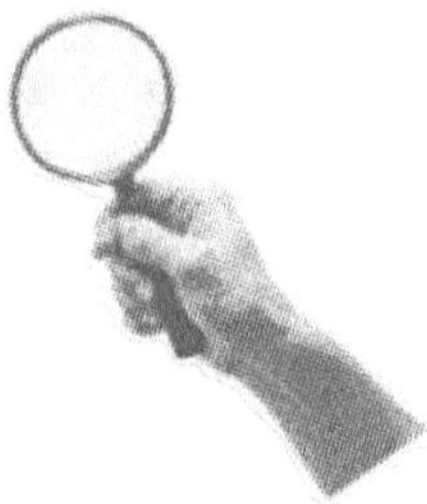

Neurodivergence, Hormones & "Why The Fuck Is Everything Harder Now?"

If you're here because your brain feels louder, foggier, more reactive, more exhausted — you're in good company. You're not late to the party. And you're not imagining this.

This book is not meant to be read cover to cover in one go. It's meant to be **used**, dipped into, ignored for a week, then returned to when you're ready.

***If you only have 5 minutes, start here:** Read the story in **Chapter 1.** Look at the **Neuro-hormonal Symptom Decoder.** Circle (or mentally note) anything that made you say *"oh... that's me."*

***If you're overwhelmed:** Go to **Chapter 4 (Sleep).** Sleep is the foundation. Everything else is harder without it.

***If your brain feels broken at work or home:** Go to **Chapter 3 (Executive Function & Capacity).** Ignore productivity culture. Focus on *capacity*, not output.

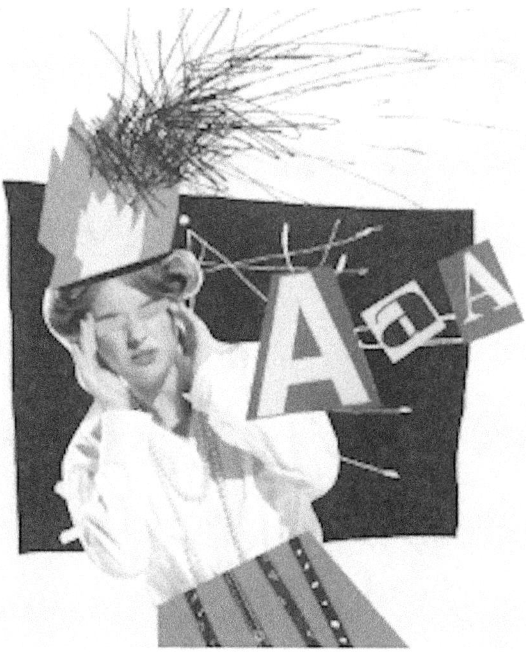

***If you feel emotionally raw, reactive, or not like yourself:**

Go to **Chapter 1 and read the reminder on pp. 32-33.** Especially if panic, rage, or dark thoughts feel new.

You do NOT have to:

*Read everything * Fix everything * Know what to do next*

You only have to take **one small step** that works for *your* nervous system, and that small step can even be finding that one account in the community resource guide in **Chapter 6** that helps you feel immediately seen.

ND + Hormonal Survival Bonus Basic Glossary

... in case you need it.

It's hard to believe that just under three years ago, I didn't have my ADHD diagnosis yet (nor was I even sure I was in menopause), and despite my kids' diagnoses, I didn't know what at least half of these terms meant. Probably, most, if I'm being completely honest. If you are new to all of this, there may be a fair amount of terminology that you're unfamiliar with. It's an additional resource I created and wanted to include with you in mind, and it's mostly non-clinical, regular person language, not comprehensive, because we're already overwhelmed enough without needing another glossary for this glossary! I hope it helps. But...

Before you skim these definitions/descriptions, I would like to take a moment to refer you back to the **medical and legal disclaimer** you may have skipped at the beginning of this book because you have ADHD.

While this glossary doesn't even remotely cover the vastness of topics of neurodivergence and hormones (whether directly or tangentially related), nor are my definitions scientifically approved LOL, it exists primarily to help newbies in particular get the gist. It's a place to start to enhance your knowledge, better understand your body and brain, as well as augment your ability to advocate for yourself. Knowledge is power, and humor heals, so you get a "two-for" with some of these descriptions. What a deal!

What this glossary **is NOT: a substitute for individualized, professional medical advice, diagnosis, or treatment.**

So again: Always consult your own healthcare provider before starting, changing, or stopping any medication, hormone therapy, supplement, exercise program, or nutrition plan—especially if you have complex health needs or take other medications.

Remember: This book is for informational, educational, and supportive purposes only. It's designed to help you feel less alone and more prepared, not to replace your doctor, specialist, or therapist.

That said: If you have questions, concerns, new or worsening symptoms, or a medical emergency, contact your qualified health professional immediately. If you think you're experiencing a medical emergency, dial your country's emergency number (like 911 in the US) right now.

1. Neurodivergent Conditions, Traits & Terms

ADHD (Attention-Deficit/Hyperactivity Disorder): A neurodevelopmental brain wiring that makes focus, planning, and impulse control feel like trying to herd caffeinated cats. Not a moral failing, not just "too much coffee." Definitely NOT a trend.

Allostatic Load: The wear and tear your body takes from chronic stress, discrimination, and surviving in a world not built for you. It's why you're exhausted, not weak.

Auditory Processing Disorder (APD): Your ears work, but your brain scrambles the messages. "Did you say 'cat' or 'hat'?" Crowded rooms are hell. No, I'm not deaf. My brain just needs an extra 10 seconds to process what you just said to me. Thank you for your patience. —The MGMT.

Autism (Autism Spectrum Disorder, ASD): A lifelong brain difference affecting how you process the world. Social rules? Not always obvious. Sensory stuff? Turned up to eleven. It's not a disease, and it's definitely not a tragedy. It's a neurotype, and the world we live in can absolutely disable you, you are not disordered: the system is.

AuDHD: ADHD + Autism. Seems like a "two-for-one" combo platter, but more accurately, it's its own thing, even if AuDHD is not technically a diagnosis. You're out here hacking two competing operating systems with one processor. You are "Both, and" incarnate.

Doom Pile: A term many of us use for the slow build-up of unfinished tasks—laundry baskets left full, unopened mail, papers stacked in corners, to-do lists that never shrink. It's not laziness or lack of care. It's what happens when executive dysfunction and hormonal shifts collide, making once-manageable chores feel insurmountable.

Dyscalculia: A learning difference that makes understanding and working with numbers difficult. Often called "number dyslexia," it means your brain just isn't wired for math. Simple tasks like splitting a restaurant bill, reading a clock without hands, or remembering phone numbers can turn into an everyday tragi-comedy.

Dysgraphia: A learning difference that makes the physical act of writing feel like a brutal Olympic sport. People with dysgraphia often know exactly what they want to say, but translating those thoughts onto paper involves a messy, exhausting war between their brain, hand, and pencil. Think of it as your brain's internal autocorrect having a total meltdown. You have brilliant, Shakespearean thoughts in your head, but the moment you try to write them down, your hand channel-surfs and produces hieroglyphics that even an cryptographer couldn't decode.

Dyslexia: —or as I lovingly call it—Dylsexia ... A historically very misunderstood reading/writing brain difference where "one-size-fits-all" types of instruction may have made you "suck" at school. Dyslexia makes reading, spelling, and processing written language trickier and basically means the brain has its own unique layout for language. The ultimate irony? It is a hard word to actually spell.

Dyspraxia: A brain difference affecting movement, coordination, and planning physical actions. If you've ever tripped over nothing, spilled your drink, or struggled with handwriting, you know the drill.

Executive Dysfunction: When your brain's CEO is off the clock. Planning, organizing, starting or finishing things? Suddenly impossible. Not laziness—just faulty wiring.

Imposter Syndrome: The unshakeable feeling that you're a fraud, even if you're crushing it. If you're anxiously awaiting the

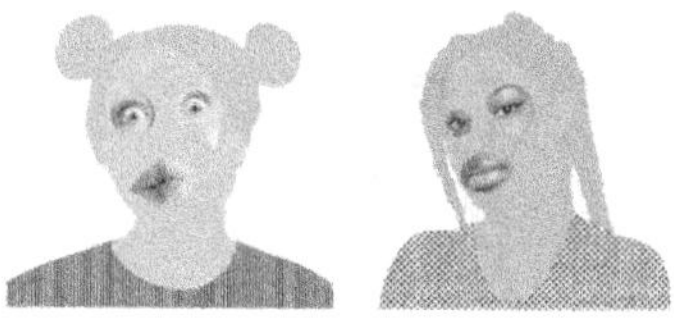

horrifying moment when someone "dramatically exposes" you, welcome to the club.

Interoception: Your body's built-in alert system that tells your brain what's going on inside. It's that voice inside you screaming, "You need to pee!," "I need coffee NOW," or warning you that those tacos were a terrible idea. Think of it as your biological Wi-Fi, constantly sending status reports about your organs, heart rate, and gut straight to your brain.

Masking: Pretending to be "normal" to avoid judgement, conflict, or drama. Exhausting, soul-sucking, and sometimes the only way to survive. But long-term? It'll burn you out.

Neurodivergent (ND): A catch-all term for anyone whose brain isn't playing by the neurotypical rulebook—think ADHD, autism, dyslexia, OCD, dyspraxia, PTSD, and so much more.

Neurodiverse: A description for any group with a mix of neurotypes (NT and ND). If everyone's the same, it's not diverse. The goal is more brains, not more sameness.

OCD (Obsessive-Compulsive Disorder): NOT "being super tidy." It's a brain glitch that causes intrusive, anxiety-driven thoughts and/or compulsive rituals. It's exhausting, not quirky, and often very dark and lonely. Remember: you are not your thoughts.

Pathologizing: Turning a normal difference or behavior into a "problem" or "disease" because it doesn't fit the mainstream narrative. Pro Tip: It's not always the person who needs to change.

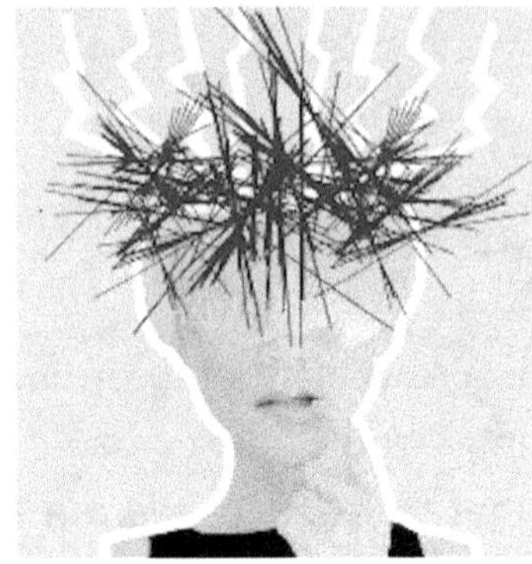

Proprioception: Your body's built-in GPS. It's the "sixth sense" that subconsciously tracks where your arms and legs are in space, letting you walk without staring at your feet and touch your nose with your eyes closed—saving you from accidentally poking yourself in the eye. Unless you have ADHD, and yours sucks like mine does. Miss your mouth constantly when you eat and drink? Run into door frames when entering rooms? Yeah, that's your proprioception basically giving you the finger.

Rejection Sensitivity Dysphoria (RSD): A lightning-fast, gut-punch reaction to even the idea of rejection or criticism. It's not "overreacting" — it's your nervous system going DEFCON 1.

Sensory Overload: When sounds, lights, smells, or even someone's breath on your neck feel like a five-alarm fire. The ND brain is a high-sensitivity instrument.

Sensory Processing Disorder (SPD): Your brain can't filter out or prioritize sensory info. Socks feel like sandpaper, tags are torture, and crowds are the ninth circle of hell.

Time Blindness: No sense of time passing, deadlines sneak attack you, and the concept of "soon" is basically theoretical. A hallmark of ADHD (and burnout).

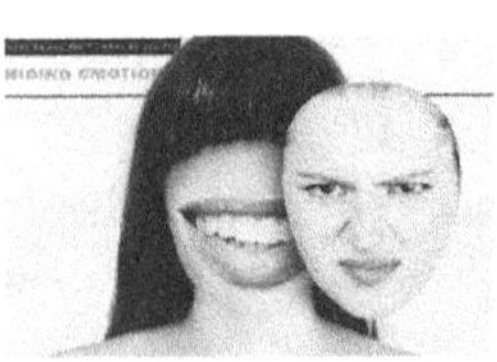

Unmasking: Dropping the act, letting your weird shine, and refusing to fake "fine." Scary as hell, but worth it.

2. Hormones, Menopause, & Related Treatments

Bioidentical Hormones: Hormones made to be chemically identical to what your body once made naturally. Often hyped, sometimes misunderstood, a viable option for many.

Estrogen: The headliner hormone for anyone born with ovaries. Declines = chaos. Affects mood, memory, skin, sex, sleep, and sanity. In short, EVERYTHING.

Gender Affirming Hormone Therapy (GAHT): A medical treatment that uses hormones (estrogen or testosterone) or blockers to align physical characteristics with a person's gender identity. It improves mental well-being and reduces gender dysphoria. While some changes are permanent, others are reversible. (Johns Hopkins, 2024)

Genitourinary Syndrome of Menopause (GSM): a cluster of symptoms affecting the genital tissues + lower urinary tract resulting from estrogen depletion. Symptoms may include dryness, irritation/itchiness down there + changes in tissue texture and elasticity; urinary tract issues may include urgency, frequency, and recurrent infections; and, in some cases, pain during sex or intimate contact. GSM can affect daily life well beyond sexual function. Sitting, cycling, and general physical comfort may all be impacted. (Firefox Allen, 2026)

Hormone Replacement Therapy (HRT): More recently referred to now as MHT, these medications are designed to replace what peri / menopause stole (estrogen, progesterone, testosterone). A life-saver for some, controversial for others. Not one-size-fits-all.

Hot Flashes / Hot Flushes: That sudden, rogue wave of volcanic heat that rolls over you (face, neck, chest), sometimes with sweating & a racing heart. Common in peri/menopause. Some say "flashes," others "flushes" — same chaos, different continents. Temperature dysregulation with an annoying twist.

Menopause: For some, it's the anniversary of your last period, but technically, it's the cessation of ovarian function. But the symptoms? They're here for the after-party. Can be surgically uninvited as well if you have your ovaries removed.

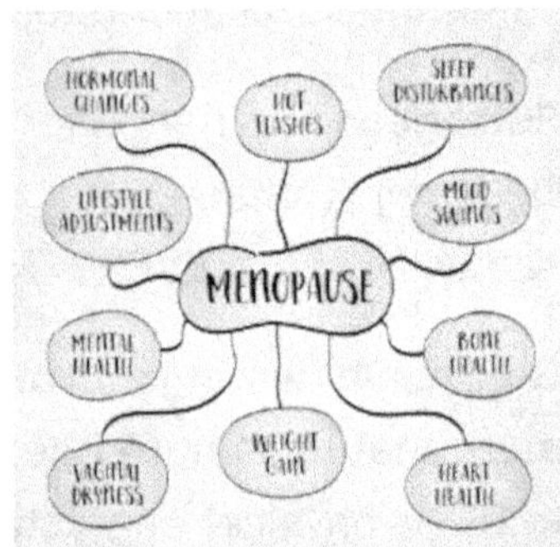

Menopausal Hormone Therapy (MHT): The more up-to-date term for HRT, specifically relating to menopause. Same hot flashes, fancier name.

Oophorectomy: The surgical removal of the ovaries, which induces immediate menopause/menopause-like symptoms

Perimenopause: The hormonal rollercoaster before menopause. Periods get weird, moods get weirder, and your body starts "beta testing" menopause years in advance.

Progesterone: The peacekeeper hormone. Drops mean sleep gets dicey, anxiety ticks up, and PMS becomes a full-time job.

Testosterone: Nope, it's not just for men. This human hormone drives libido, muscle, motivation, and mood. Declines = "where did my energy go?"

3. Neurotransmitters, Stress, & Brain Chemistry

Cortisol: The stress hormone. Great when you need to outrun a bear, terrible when you're just trying to sleep. Chronic high cortisol = body aches, brain fog, rage.

Dopamine: The brain's hype person—reward, motivation, focus. Low dopamine = apathy, forgetfulness, endless scrolling, no fucks to give.

Executive Function: The brain's control center for getting shit done—planning, prioritizing, switching gears, and remembering why you walked into the kitchen.

Norepinephrine: The "wired and tired" often neglected middle sister hormone. Everyone loves to rant and rave about serotonin and dopamine, but norepinephrine controls alertness, focus, and stress response. Too much = anxious. Too little = can't get moving.

Serotonin: The mood stabilizer. Drops = anxiety, sadness, rage crying at commercials.

Working Memory: Your brain's sticky note—temporarily holds info you need NOW (like phone numbers or directions). With ND + hormone chaos, it's less "sticky note" and more "greased slide."

4. Diagnosis & Treatment

Amphetamine/Dextroamphetamine: A combo central nervous system (CNS) stimulant medication primarily used to treat ADHD (and narcolepsy). It works by increasing neurotransmitter levels (dopamine and norepinephrine) to improve focus and control impulses. The most common brand is **Adderall.**

CBT (Cognitive Behavioral Therapy): A structured, short-term, and goal-oriented talk therapy that helps people identify and change negative or irrational thought patterns and behaviors. It is highly effective for treating anxiety, depression, phobias, and addiction by focusing on present-day challenges. For Autism and ADHD that often get misdiagnosed as "just" anxiety? Not so much.

DBT (Dialectical Behavior Therapy): A structured, evidence-based psychotherapy designed to help people manage intensely emotional experiences, improve relationships, and reduce self-destructive behaviors. It combines cognitive-behavioral techniques with mindfulness, focusing on balancing emotional acceptance with positive behavioral change.

DSM-5 (Diagnostic and Statistical Manual of Mental Disorders, Fifth Edition): The official playbook for mental health diagnoses in the U.S.—sometimes helpful, sometimes limiting, always up for debate. If you don't feel like having your neurotype pathologized as "disorder," don't read this manual. Not that you would if you're not a medical/mental health provider. That said, if you need real world accommodations for work and/or school as well as access to medication for treatment, you may gain a certain appreciation for this diagnostic tool.

EMDR (Eye Movement Desensitization and Reprocessing): An effective, evidence-based psychotherapy designed to alleviate distress from traumatic memories and PTSD. It involves focusing on traumatic memories while experiencing bilateral stimulation (like side-to-side eye movements), helping the brain reprocess memories to reduce their emotional charge.

ERP (Exposure and Response Prevention): The primary, first-line treatment for OCD. It involves gradually exposing you to triggers (obsessions) while asking you to actively resist the urge to perform compulsive rituals. This helps desensitize you to the anxiety and breaks the OCD feedback loop.

Exposure Therapy: A highly effective psychological treatment that helps individuals confront their fears and break the cycle of avoidance. By systematically and gradually exposing patients to feared objects, situations, or memories in a safe environment, it retrains the brain to reduce distress and build tolerance.

ICD-11 (International Classification of Diseases, 11th Revision): The World Health Organization's (WHO) global standard for health information, providing a common language for diseases and health conditions, with a major update for mental, behavioral, and neurodevelopmental disorders released in 2024 as the Clinical Descriptions and Diagnostic Requirements (CDDR). Do not recommend for book clubs or your next beach vacation read!

Nonstimulant Medication (for ADHD): The alternative class of ADHD meds for those who can't (or don't want to) use stimulants. Includes options like atomoxetine, guanfacine, and clonidine. Often gentler, sometimes slower-acting, but game-changers for the right brain.

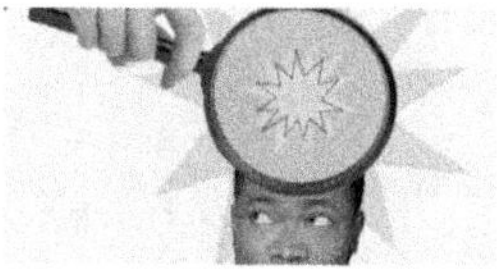

Stimulant Medication (for ADHD): First-line treatment for ADHD, these meds (like methylphenidate and amphetamines) crank up dopamine and norepinephrine in the brain. For most, they boost focus, motivation, and impulse control — not a "quick fix," but actual, evidence-based medicine. Not everyone reacts the same, so it's about finding your personal groove.

Lisdexamfetamine: A central nervous system (CNS) stimulant indicated for treating ADHD (and moderate-to-severe binge eating disorder (BED) in adults. **Vyvanse** is a well-known name brand.

Methylphenidate: A central nervous system (CNS) stimulant used to treat ADHD (and narcolepsy). It works by increasing dopamine and norepinephrine levels in the brain to improve focus, reduce impulsivity, and promote wakefulness. Major brand names include **Concerta, Ritalin, Daytrana, and Quillivant XR.** Pro-tip (and actual scientific fact): this is not street Meth. Crystal meth is illegal and will kill you. Methylphenidate is one of the gold standards of ADHD treatment, and not only is it legal, it might just save your life. Reminder: I'm not a medical professional. Consult yours about any and all medications and treatment plans.

Sources Cited and Consulted

1. Menopause endocrinology, hormone therapy, and core clinical care

• **American College of Obstetricians and Gynecologists.** (2023). Compounded bioidentical menopausal hormone therapy. ACOG Clinical Consensus No. 6. *Obstetrics & Gynecology, 142*(5), 1266–1273. https://doi.org/10.1097/AOG.0000000000005397

• **Elggren, C. W. et al.** (2026). Testosterone Replacement Therapy in Women Is Associated with Improved Symptom Burden and Favorable Biomarker Changes: A Retrospective Observational Study. *Journal of Personalized Medicine, 16*(5), 231. https://doi.org/10.3390/jpm16050231

• **European Society of Endocrinology.** (2025, October 22). *Press release: ESE announces new Clinical Practice Guideline for Management and Evaluation of Menopause and the Perimenopause.* https://www.ese-hormones.org/news/press-release-ese-announces-new-clinical-practice-guideline-for-management-and-evaluation-of-menopause-and-the-perimenopause/

• **Gompel, A., & Simcock, R.** (2026). Menopausal hormone treatment and breast cancer. The Lancet Diabetes & Endocrinology, *14*(3), 259–274. https://doi.org/10.1016/S2213-8587(25)00394-8

• **Gravelsins, L. L., & Galea, L. A. M.** (2025). One size does not fit all: how type of menopause and hormone therapy matters for brain health. *The British Journal of Psychiatry, 226*(6), 369–382. https://doi.org/10.1192/bjp.2025.52

• **Johansen, N., Lindén Hirschberg, A., & Moen, M. H.** (2020). The role of testosterone in menopausal hormone treatment. What is the evidence? *Acta Obstetricia et Gynecologica Scandinavica*, 99(8), 966–969. 10.1111/aogs.13819 https://doi.org/10.1111/aogs.13819

• **Johns Hopkins Medicine.** (2024, October 25). *Gender-affirming hormone therapy (GAHT).* https://www.hopkinsmedicine.org/health/treatment-tests-and-therapies/gender-affirming-hormone-therapy-gaht

• **Kim, Y., Cho, M. K. et al.** (2025). Publication Committee on Clinical Guidelines of the Korean Society of Menopause. The 2025 Menopausal Hormone Therapy Guidelines - Korean Society of Menopause. *Journal of menopausal medicine, 31*(2), 53–84. https://doi.org/10.6118/jmm.25103

• **Krewson, C.** (2025, December 21). *Nonhormonal therapies transform menopause care in 2025. Contemporary OB/GYN.* https://www.contemporaryobgyn.net/view/nonhormonal-therapies-transform-menopause-care-in-2025
• **Mikkelsen A. P., Bergholt, T., Lideg, Ø., Scheller, N. M.** (2026). Menopausal hormone therapy and long term mortality: nationwide, register based cohort study *BMJ* ; 392 :e085998 https://doi.org/10.1136/bmj-2025-085998
• **North American Menopause Society.** (2024). *Genitourinary syndrome of menopause: Current approaches. Menopause, 31*(2), 119–128. https://doi.org/10.1097/GME.0000000000002292
• **North American Menopause Society.** (2024). *Position statement: Hormone therapy. Menopause, 31*(2), 112–123. https://doi.org/10.1097/GME.0000000000002291
• **Santoro, N., & Neal-Perry, G.** (2024). *Menopause: The role of hormone testing. Journal of Clinical Endocrinology & Metabolism, 109*(2), 445–452. https://doi.org/10.1210/clinem/dgad673
• **Talaulikar V.** (2022). Menopause transition: Physiology and symptoms. *Best Practice & Research Clinical Obstetrics & Gynaecology*, 81, 3–7. https://doi.org/10.1016/j.bpobgyn.2022.03.003
• **Tan, D. A., & Dayu, A. R. B.** (2022). *Menopausal hormone therapy: why we should no longer be afraid of the breast cancer risk. Climacteric: The Journal of the International Menopause Society, 25*(4), 362–368. https://doi.org/10.1080/13697137.2022.2035711

2. Brain, executive function, cognition, and neurobiology

• **Diamond, A.** (2013). *Executive functions. Annual Review of Psychology, 64*, 135–168. https://doi.org/10.1146/annurev-psych-113011-143750
• **Faubion, S. S., Santoro, N., & Warren, M. P.** (2023). *Menopause and the brain: The impact of estrogen deficiency. Climacteric, 26*(1), 21–29. https://doi.org/10.1080/13697137.2022.2116200
• **Luine V. N.** (2014). Estradiol and cognitive function: past, present and future. *Hormones and behavior, 66*(4), 602–618. https://doi.org/10.1016/j.yhbeh.2014.08.011
• **Maki, P. M., & Sundermann, E.** (2021). *Hormone therapy and cognitive function. Neurobiology of Aging, 99*, 81–87. https://doi.org/10.1016/j.neurobiolaging.2020.05.011
• **Reuter-Lorenz, P. A., & Cappell, K. A.** (2023). *The neurobiology of aging & executive dysfunction. Annual Review of Psychology, 74*, 139–166. https://doi.org/10.1146/annurev-psych-070222-030303

- **Russell, J. K., Jones, C. K., & Newhouse, P. A.** (2019). *The role of estrogen in brain and cognitive aging. Neurotherapeutics, 16*(3), 649–665. https://doi.org/10.1007/s13311-019-00766-9
- **Shanmugan, S., & Epperson, C. N.** (2014). *Estrogen and the prefrontal cortex: Towards a new understanding of estrogen's effects on executive functions in the menopause transition. Human Brain Mapping, 35*, 847–865. https://doi.org/10.1002/hbm.22218
- **Snyder, H. R., Miyake, A., & Hankin, B. L.** (2015). *Executive function impairments & psychopathology. Development and Psychopathology, 27*(4 Pt 2), 1399–1414. https://doi.org/10.1017/S0954579415000883
- **Sood, R., Kuhle, C. L., Kapoor, E., Thielen, J. M., Frohmader, K. S., Mara, K. C., & Faubion, S. S.** (2019). Association of mindfulness and stress with menopausal symptoms in midlife women. *Climacteric, 22*(4), 377–382. https://doi.org/10.1080/13697137.2018.1551344
- **Weber, M. T., Maki, P. M., & McDermott, M. P.** (2014). Cognition and mood in perimenopause: a systematic review and meta-analysis. *The Journal of steroid biochemistry and molecular biology, 142*, 90–98. https://doi.org/10.1016/j.jsbmb.2013.06.001
- **Yadav, P., Yadav, S., Vedururu, S. S., & Kumari, G.** (2025). A Standardized *Asparagus Racemosus* Root Extract Improves Hormonal Balance and Menstrual Health and Reduces Vasomotor Symptoms in Perimenopausal Women: A Randomized, Double-Blind, Placebo-Controlled Study. *Journal of the American Nutrition Association, 44*(8), 754–764. https://doi.org/10.1080/27697061.2025.2510474
- **Zachry, J. E., Nolan, S. O., Brady, L. J., Kelly, S. J., Siciliano, C. A., & Calipari, E. S.** (2021). *Sex differences in dopamine release regulation in the striatum. Neuropsychopharmacology, 46*, 491–499. https://doi.org/10.1038/s41386-020-00915-1

3. Sleep, circadian rhythm, and sensory environment

- **Cho, Y., et al.** (2016). *Artificial light at night and human health. Chronobiology International, 33*(9), 1087–1100. https://doi.org/10.1080/07420528.2016.1183473
- **Edinger, J. D. & Means, M. K.** (2005). *CBT for primary insomnia. Clinical Psychology Review, 25*(5), 539–558. https://doi.org/10.1016/j.cpr.2005.04.003
- **Faraut, B. et al.** (2015). *Napping: A public health issue. Sleep Medicine Reviews, 22*, 85–100. https://doi.org/10.1016/j.smrv.2014.11.003
- **Gao, C., Zhao, X., Qiu, Z. & Duan, Z.** (2022). *Sound interventions for improving sleep. Sensors, 22*(3), 976. https://doi.org/10.3390/s22030976

• **Kravitz, H. M., Joffe, H. & Crawford, S. L.** (2023). *Sleep disturbance and menopause: Clinical considerations. Nature Reviews Endocrinology, 19*(2), 91–106. https://doi.org/10.1038/s41574-022-00796-8
• **Lustenberger, C. et al.** (2022). *Acoustic stimulation during sleep. Communications Medicine, 2*, 16. https://doi.org/10.1038/s43856-022-00116-0
• **Mednick, S., Nakayama, K. & Stickgold, R.** (2003). *Sleep-dependent learning. Nature Neuroscience, 6*(7), 697–698. https://doi.org/10.1038/nn1078
• **Morin, C. M. & Benca, R.** (2012). *Chronic insomnia. The Lancet, 379*(9821), 1129–1141. https://doi.org/10.1016/S0140-6736(11)60750-2
• **Okamoto-Mizuno, K. & Mizuno, K.** (2012). *Thermal environment and sleep. Journal of Physiological Anthropology, 31*(1), 14. https://doi.org/10.1186/1880-6805-31-14
• **Peled, R. et al.** (2023). *Weighted blankets and sleep. Frontiers in Psychiatry, 14*, 1159845. https://doi.org/10.3389/fpsyt.2023.1159845
• **Roehrs, T. & Roth, T.** (2022). *Sleep and neurobehavioral functioning. Neurotherapeutics, 19*(1), 25–39. https://doi.org/10.1007/s13311-021-01153-1
• **Saxbe, D. E. & Repetti, R.** (2010). *No Place Like Home: Home Tours Correlate With Daily Patterns of Mood and Cortisol. Personality and Social Psychology Bulletin, 36*(1), 71–81. https://doi.org/10.1177/0146167209352864
• **Vitiello, M. V. & Rybarczyk, B.** (2022). *Sleep disruption in menopause. Sleep Medicine Clinics, 17*(3), 365–376. https://doi.org/10.1016/j.jsmc.2022.04.007
• **Wang, C., Ong, J. L. & Chee, M. W. L.** (2023). *Acoustic stimulation and memory. Neuroscience & Biobehavioral Reviews, 149*, 105162. https://doi.org/10.1016/j.neubiorev.2023.105162

4. Neurodivergence across hormones and hormonal transitions

• **ADDitude Magazine.** (2024). *Sex hormones and ADHD.* https://www.additudemag.com/sex-hormones-adhd-inattention-emotional-dysregulation-impulsivity/
• **ADDitude Magazine.** (2025, February). *ADHD impairment peaks in menopause, according to ADDitude reader survey.*
• **Bjelland, J.** (2025, September). *Survey results: Perimenopause and menopause in sensitive and neurodivergent women.* Julie Bjelland. https://www.juliebjelland.com/hsp-blog/survey-results-perimenopause-and-menopause-in-sensitive-and-neurodivergent-women-by-julie-bjelland-lmft
• **Brady, M. J., Jenkins, C. A., Gamble-Turner, J. M., Moseley, R. L.,**

Janse van Rensburg, M. & Matthews, R. J. (2024). "A perfect storm": Autistic experiences of menopause and midlife. *Autism, 28*(6), 1405–1418.

• **Camara, B., Padoin, C. & Bolea, B.** (2022). *Relationship between sex hormones, reproductive stages and ADHD: A systematic review. Archives of Women's Mental Health, 25*, 1–8. https://doi.org/10.1007/s00737-021-01181-w

• **Chapman, L., Gupta, K., Hunter, M. S. & Dommett, E. J.** (2025). Examining the Link Between ADHD Symptoms and Menopausal Experiences. *Journal of Attention Disorders, 29*(14), 1263-1277. https://doi.org/10.1177/10870547251355006

• **Chronis-Tuscano A.** (2022). *ADHD in girls and women: a call to action – reflections on Hinshaw et al. (2021). J Child Psychol Psychiatry, 63*(4), 497–499.

• **Dorani, F., Bijlenga, D., Beekman, A., van Someren, E. & Kooij, J.** (2021). *Prevalence of hormone-related mood disorder symptoms in women with ADHD. Journal of Psychiatric Research, 133*, 10–15. https://doi.org/10.1016/j.jpsychires.2020.12.005

• **Elektra Health.** (2021). *Neurodiversity and menopause: Emerging evidence.*

• **Epperson, C. N. et al.** (2015). New onset executive function difficulties at menopause: a possible role for lisdexamfetamine. *Psychopharmacology, 232*(16), 3091–3100. https://doi.org/10.1007/s00213-015-3953-7

• **Groenman, A. P., Torenvliet, C., Radhoe, T. A., Agelink van Rentergem, J. A. & Geurts, H. M.** (2022). *Menstruation and menopause in autistic adults: Periods of importance? Autism, 26*, 1563–1572. https://doi.org/10.1177/13623613211059721

• **Hinshaw, S. P., Nguyen, P. T., O'Grady, S. M. & Rosenthal, E. A.** (2022). *Annual research review: Attention-deficit/hyperactivity disorder in girls and women: underrepresentation, longitudinal processes, and key directions. J Child Psychol Psychiatry, 63*(4), 484–496.

• **Hutson, P. & Hutson, J.** (2025). *Premenopausal transition in neurodivergent women with musculoskeletal syndromes: Mechanisms, risks, and neuroinclusive therapeutics. International Journal of Human Research and Social Science Studies, 2*(9), 696–712. https://doi.org/10.55677/ijhrsss/14-2025-Vol02I9

• **Jakobsdóttir Smári, U. et al.** (2025). *Perimenopausal symptoms in women with and without ADHD: A population-based cohort study. European Psychiatry, 68*(1), e133. https://doi.org/10.1192/j.eurpsy.2025.10101

• **Jenkins, C. A., Moseley, R. L., Matthews, R. J., van Rensburg, M. J., Gamble-Turner, J. M. & Brady, M. J.** (2024). "Struggling for Years": An international survey on Autistic experiences of menopause. *Neurodiversity, 2*. https://doi.org/10.1177/27546330241299З

- **Karavidas, M. & de Visser, R. O.** (2022). "It's Not Just in My Head, and It's Not Just Irrelevant": Autistic Negotiations of Menopausal Transitions. *Journal of autism and developmental disorders, 52*(3), 1143–1155. https://doi.org/10.1007/s10803-021-05010-y
- **Kelly ,C. A., Kelly, C. & Taylor, R.** (2024). *Review of the psychosocial consequences of attention deficit hyperactivity disorder (ADHD) in females. European Journal of Medical and Health Sciences, 6*(1), 10–20.
- **Kooij, J. J. S. et al.** (2025). *Research advances and future directions in female ADHD. Frontiers in Global Women's Health, 6*, 1613628. https://doi.org/10.3389/fgwh.2025.1613628
- **Krebs, K. & Donnellan-Fernandez, R.** (2025). *Integrative literature review – the impact of ADHD across women's lifespan. BMC Women's Health, 25*, 593. https://doi.org/10.1186/s12905-025-04123-1
- **Moseley, R. L., Gamble-Turner, J. M., Kim, E. & Spencer, C.** (2026). Autism, ADHD and the menopause. *Post Reproductive Health*, 1–11. https://doi.org/10.1080/20533691.2026.2631222
- **Myla Health.** (n.d.). *ADHD, ASD & menopause.* https://www.mylahealth.co.uk/adhd-menopause
- **Newson, L.** (2023). *Menopause and neurodiversity: Overlapping challenges. Post Reproductive Health, 29*(1), 44–52. https://doi.org/10.1177/20533691231119349
- **Pines, A.** (2016). Midlife ADHD in women: Any relevance to menopause? *Climacteric*, 19(5), 423–425.
- **Roberts, B., Eisenlohr-Moul, T. & Martel, M. M.** (2018). *Reproductive steroids and ADHD symptoms across the menstrual cycle. Psychoneuroendocrinology, 88*, 105–114. https://doi.org/10.1016/j.psyneuen.2017.11.015
- **Sehinson, C. E.** (2025, June 25). *Perimenopause and neurodivergence (part 1).* https://www.claireelizasehinson.com/blog/perimenopause-and-neurodivergence
- **SI St Albans and District.** (2025, October 28). *Mental health challenges with ADHD and menopause – Dr Samantha Hiew.* https://sigbi.org/st-albans-and-district/2025/mentalhealth25/
- **Wallin, K., Alehagen, S., Hanberger, L., Lundell, I.W. & Hultsjö, S.** (2024). *Sexual and reproductive health in young women with ADHD from the view of health care professionals. BMC Womens Health, 24*(1), 389.
- **West, S.** (2025). *Body-identical HRT: Why it matters for neurodivergent women.* https://www.sarahwest-adhd.com/blog/menstruacycle-neurodivergent-dwwhn

5. ADHD diagnosis, treatment, and sex/gender-informed clinical management

- **Babinski, D. E.** (2024). *Sex differences in ADHD: Review and priorities for future research. Current Psychiatry Reports, 26*, 151–156. https://doi.org/10.1007/s11920-024-01492-6
- **Cortese, S. et al.** (2021). *Comparative efficacy of ADHD medications. The Lancet Psychiatry, 8*(6), 487–498. https://doi.org/10.1016/S2215-0366(21)00095-7
- **Faraone, S. V. et al.** (2021). *ADHD. Nature Reviews Disease Primers, 7*(1), 47. https://doi.org/10.1038/s41572-021-00270-2
- **Franke, B.** (2023). *Editorial: It is time to modernize the concept of ADHD! Journal of Child Psychology and Psychiatry, 64*, 845–847. https://doi.org/10.1111/jcpp.13812
- **Kok, F. M., Groen, Y. & Führmaier, A. B. M.** (2020). *The female side of pharmacotherapy for ADHD—A systematic literature review. PLOS One, 15*(9), e0239257.
- **Kooij, J. S.** (2024). *ADHD in a women during (peri)menopause: missed diagnoses and cardiac complaints. European Psychiatry, 67*(Suppl 1), S800. https://doi.org/10.1192/j.eurpsy.2024.1666
- **Lai, M.-C., Lin, H.-Y. & Ameis, S. H.** (2022). *Towards equitable diagnoses for autism and attention-deficit/hyperactivity disorder across sexes and genders. Current Opinion in Psychiatry, 35*, 90. https://doi.org/10.1097/YCO.0000000000000770
- **National Institute for Health and Care Excellence.** (2018). *ADHD: Diagnosis and management (NG87).* https://www.nice.org.uk/guidance/ng87
- **Prevatt, F. & Yelland, S.** (2015). *ADHD coaching in college students. Journal of Attention Disorders, 19*(8), 666–677. https://doi.org/10.1177/1087054713506261
- **Rapoport, I. L. & Groenman, A. P.** (2025). *A Review of Sex and Gender Factors in Stimulant Treatment for ADHD: Knowledge Gaps and Future Directions. Journal of Attention Disorders, 29*(8), 602–616. https://doi.org/10.1177/10870547251315601
- **Wolraich, M. L. et al.** (2019). *ADHD clinical practice guideline. Pediatrics, 144*(4), e20192528. https://doi.org/10.1542/peds.2019-2528
- **Wynchank, D., de Jong, M. & Kooij, S. J. J. S.** (2025). *Practical tools for female-specific ADHD: The impact of hormonal fluctuations in clinical practice and from the literature. European Psychiatry, 69*(1), e1. https://doi.org/10.1192/j.eurpsy.2025.10120
- **Young, S. et al.** (2020). *Females with ADHD: An expert consensus statement taking a lifespan approach providing guidance for the identification

and treatment of attention-deficit/hyperactivity disorder in girls and women. BMC Psychiatry, 20, 404. https://doi.org/10.1186/s12888-020-02707-9

6. Neurodivergent midlife lived experience, masking, mental health, and sexuality

• **Aiken, C. E., Walker, A. L., Sassarini, J. & Smith, R.** (2023). *Autistic experiences of menopause: A qualitative study exploring identity, masking, and health care interactions. Autism, 27*(6), 1510–1524.
• **Bargiela, S., Steward, R. & Mandy, W.** (2020). The Female Autism Phenotype and Camouflaging: a Narrative Review.*Rev J Autism Dev Disord* **7**, 306–317. https://doi.org/10.1007/s40489-020-00197-9
• **Brady, M. J., Jenkins, C. A., Gamble-Turner, J. M., Moseley, R. L., Janse van Rensburg, M. G. & Matthews, R. J.** (2024). *"A perfect storm": Autistic experiences of menopause and midlife. Autism, 28*(6), 1405–1418. https://doi.org/10.1177/13623613241244548
• **Crockett, C., Lichtveld, G., Macdonald, R., Newson, L. & Rampling, K. J.** (2026). *Menopause and Mental Health. Advances in Therapy, 43*(1), 98–108. https://doi.org/10.1007/s12325-025-03427-w
• **Flanagan, K. & Berridge, C.** (2023). *Menopause, neurodivergence, and the limits of the biomedical model: A neuroaffirming perspective. Women's Health, 19*, 17455057231130124.
• **Hendriks, O., McIntyre, J. C., Rose, A. K., Crockett, C., Newson, L. & Saini, P.** (2025). *The mental health challenges, especially suicidality, experienced by women during perimenopause and menopause: A qualitative study. Women's Health, 21*, 17455057251338941. https://doi.org/10.1177/17455057251338941
• **Kroese, A. C. et al.** (2024). *Sexual function and neurodivergence in midlife women. Journal of Menopausal Health, 30*(1), 22–37. https://doi.org/10.1097/JMH.0000000000001357
• **Patalay, P.** (2019). *Masking in transgender and neurodivergent communities: A cross-sectional analysis of emotional labor. Transgender Health, 4*(2), 105–112. https://doi.org/10.1089/trgh.2019.0015
• **Peters, M. L. & Taylor, R. J.** (2024). *Menopause and the mental health of neurodivergent women: A biopsychosocial overview. Archives of Women's Mental Health, 27*(2), 173–186.
• **Rapisarda, F. et al.** (2021). *Masking, neurodivergence, and social health in autistic and ADHD adults. Journal of Autism and Developmental Disorders, 51*(10), 3565–3580. https://doi.org/10.1007/s10803-020-04810-3
• **Tranchitella, T.** (2023, December 1). *ADHD in women: From the dreamy-eyed*

girl in the back of the classroom to the menopausal woman who can't find her keys (again). Hormone Lab UK. https://hormonelab.co.uk/fr/blogs/blog/adhd-in-women-girl-in-classroom-to-menopausal-woman-losing-keys

7. LGBTQIA+, trans, nonbinary, and gender-affirming menopause care

- **Drysdale, K., Karasu, Y. & Watson, L.** (2026). *"Because I felt so alone": trans and gender diverse people's needs and preferences for menopausal related information and resources. International Journal of Transgender Health*, 1–14. https://doi.org/10.1080/26895269.2026.2618635
- **Firefox Allen, L.** (2026). *Genderqueer menopause: Navigating menopause for trans, gender-nonconforming, genderfluid, and other queer-bodied folx.* North Atlantic Books.
- **Gianelis, K. & Allen, L.F.** (2026). *Gender-Affirming Menopause Care: Best Practices. Clinical Journal for Nurse Practitioners in Women's Health, 3*, 33–40. https://doi.org/10.1891/CJNPWH-2025-0036
- **Glyde, T.** (2023). How can therapists and other healthcare practitioners best support and validate their queer menopausal clients? *Sexual and Relationship Therapy*, 38(4), 510–532. https://doi.org/10.1080/14681994.2021.1881770
- **Goetz, T. G. & Adams, N.** (2024). *The Transgender and Gender Diverse and Attention Deficit Hyperactivity Disorder Nexus: A Systematic Review. Journal of Gay & Lesbian Mental Health, 28*(1), 2–19. https://doi.org/10.1080/19359705.2022.2109119
- **Gravely, A. K. & Brotto, L. A.** (2026). *The non-cisgender experience of menstruation and menopause: Literature review and recommendations. Journal of Obstetrics and Gynaecology Canada, 48*(1), 103161. https://doi.org/10.1016/j.jogc.2025.103161
- **Kimber, B., Oxlad, M. & Twyford, L.** (2024). *The impact of microaggressions on the mental health of trans and gender-diverse people: A scoping review. International Journal of Transgender Health,* 0(0), 1–21. https://doi.org/10.1080/26895269.2024.2380903
- **Libby, V., Lee, M. & Liu, J. H.** (2019). *Transgender health: Hormonal management at 50 years and beyond. Maturitas, 126*, 34–37. https://doi.org/10.1016/j.maturitas.2019.04.220
- **McNeil, J., Bailey, L., Ellis, S., Morton, J. & Regan, M.** (2012). *Trans mental health study 2012.* Scottish Transgender Alliance. https://www.scottishtrans.org/trans_mh_study/
- **Plume Health.** (2022, July 26). *Understanding how testosterone can affect*

your emotions during transition. https://getplume.co/blog/understanding-how-testosterone-can-affect-your-emotions-during-transition/
• **Pyne, Y.** (2024, October 18). *Navigating perimenopause and menopause as a trans person: Challenges, insights, and support. Primary Care Research & Teaching Blog.* https://capcbristol.blogs.bristol.ac.uk/2024/10/18/navigating-perimenopause-and-menopause-as-a-trans-person-challenges-insights-and-support/
• **Scandurra, C., Mezza, F., Maldonato, N. M., Bottone, M., Bochicchio, V., Valerio, P. & Vitelli, R.** (2019). Health of non-binary and genderqueer people: A systematic review. *Frontiers in Psychology*, 10, 1453. https://doi.org/10.3389/fpsyg.2019.01453
• **Sobel, T., Derakshani, D. & Vencill, J. A.** (2024). *Menopause experiences in sexual minority women and non-binary people. Maturitas, 185*, 108007. https://doi.org/10.1016/j.maturitas.2024.108007
• **Tarquini, L.** (Host). (n.d.). *Menopause from a transgender perspective* (Season 3, Episode 6) [Audio podcast episode]. In *The Menopause Space.* RSS.com. https://rss.com/podcasts/the-menopause-space/1921633/
• **Thrower, E., Bretherton, I., Pang, K. C., Zajac, J. D. & Cheung, A. S.** (2020). *Prevalence of autism spectrum disorder and attention-deficit hyperactivity disorder amongst individuals with gender dysphoria: A systematic review. Journal of Autism and Developmental Disorders, 50*(3), 695–706. https://doi.org/10.1007/s10803-019-04298-1
• **Toze, M. & Westwood, S.** (2025). *Experiences of menopause among non-binary and trans people. International Journal of Transgender Health, 26*(2), 447–458. https://doi.org/10.1080/26895269.2024.2389924
• **Westwood, S.** (2025). *Lesbian, gay, bisexual, transgender and queer (LGBTQ+) menopause: Literature review, knowledge gaps and research agenda. Health, 29*(4), 468–488. https://doi.org/10.1177/13634593241270923
• **Windt, I. K., Mullens, A. B., Debattista, J., Stanners, M. & Brömdal, A.** (2024). *Developing a gender affirming health response for trans and gender diverse Australians: A qualitative study. International Journal of Transgender Health*, 1–18. https://doi.org/10.1080/26895269.2024.2374007

8. Relationships, social support, and relational wellbeing in midlife

• **Brown, S. L. & Lin, I.-F.** (2023). *Divorce after midlife. American Sociological Review, 88*(2), 305–332. https://doi.org/10.1177/00031224231162348
• **Cacioppo, J. T. et al.** (2015). *Neuroendocrinology of social isolation.*

Annual Review of Psychology, 66, 733–767. https://doi.org/10.1146/annurev-psych-010814-015240
• **McEwen, B. S.** (2023). *Social relationships and the brain. Nature Reviews Neuroscience, 24*(2), 109–122. https://doi.org/10.1038/s41583-022-00722-y
• **Parish, S. J., Faubion, S. S., Weinberg, M., Bernick, B. & Mirkin, S.** (2019). *The MATE survey: men's perceptions and attitudes towards menopause and their role in partners' menopausal transition. Menopause, 26*(10), 1110–1116. https://doi.org/10.1097/GME.0000000000001373
• **Trujillo, L.** (2026, January 5). *Welcome to the "menodivorce": Why women aren't sweating marriage in a sea of hot flashes. USA Today.* https://www.usatoday.com/story/life/health-wellness/2025/08/14/divorce-women-perimenopause-menopause/85622804007/
• **Tuncer, S. K., Karakurt, P., Özdemir, S. & Bilgin, S.** (2026). *The relationship between spousal support and quality of life in postmenopausal women: a cross-sectional study. Revista da Associacao Medica Brasileira (1992), 71*(12), e20251068. https://doi.org/10.1590/1806-9282.20251068
• **Williams, D. R. & Anderson, N. B.** (2022). *Social support and health in adulthood. Annual Review of Public Health, 43*, 423–441. https://doi.org/10.1146/annurev-publhealth-052020-020932
• **Willmott, L. & Bentley, E.** (2015). Exploring the Lived-Experience of Limerence: A Journey toward Authenticity. *The Qualitative Report, 20*(1), 20-38. https://doi.org/10.46743/2160-3715/2015.1420
• **Yildirim, F., Duman, N. B. & Kulakaç, Ö.** (2023). *The Effect of Menopause on the Sexual Functions and Marital Adjustment of the Spouses. Journal of Mid-life Health, 14*(3), 170–175. https://doi.org/10.4103/jmh.jmh_90_23

9. Race, racism, culture, and structural inequities in menopause

• **Alloy Health.** (n.d.). *Unique challenges faced by Black and Native women during menopause | Dr. Judith Joseph* [Video]. YouTube. https://www.youtube.com/watch?v=zv4GwwrAni8
• **Amalka.** (2025, October 22). *Menopause: The intersection of race, neurodivergence, and mental health. Medium.* https://medium.com/@amalka6/menopause-the-intersection-of-race-neurodivergence-and-mental-health-b455c7d69976
• **Blanken, A., Gibson, C. J., Li, Y., Huang, A. J., Byers, A. L., Maguen, S., Inslicht, S. & Seal, K.** (2022). *Racial/ethnic disparities in the diagnosis and management of menopause symptoms among midlife women veterans. Menopause, 29*(7), 877–882. https://doi.org/10.1097/GME.0000000000001978

• **Carothers, C., Lee, K. A. & Matthews, K. A.** (2024). *The association of race, ethnicity, and socioeconomic status with the severity of menopause symptoms in 68,864 women. Menopause, 31*(6), 643–652.

• **Charles, R. A. & Chichaya, T. F.** (2025). *A Qualitative Exploration of the Lived Experience of Menopause Among Black Women in the United Kingdom. Public Health Challenges, 4*(4), e70168. https://doi.org/10.1002/puh2.70168

• **Gold, E. B., Sternfeld, B. & Kelsey, J. L.** (2023). *Race, social context, and psychosocial well-being in midlife women: Lessons from SWAN. Journal of Health and Social Behavior, 64*(2), 198–213.

• **Harlow, S. D., Burnett-Bowie, S. M., Greendale, G. A., Avis, N. E., Reeves, A. N., Richards, T. R. & Lewis, T. T.** (2022). *Disparities in Reproductive Aging and Midlife Health between Black and White women: The Study of Women's Health Across the Nation (SWAN). Women's Midlife Health, 8*(1), 3. https://doi.org/10.1186/s40695-022-00073-y

• **Im, E. O., Seung Hee Lee & Chee, W.** (2010). *Subethnic differences in the menopausal symptom experience of Asian American midlife women. Journal of Transcultural Nursing, 21*(2), 123–133. https://doi.org/10.1177/1043659609357639

• **Krohe, M., Price, P. D., Simeone, D., Gagne, L., King, D. D. & Seele, P. C.** (2025). *A survey to understand the experience, perceptions, and stigma around menopause among African American women. Preventive Medicine Reports, 61*, 103341. https://doi.org/10.1016/j.pmedr.2025.103341

• **Lewis Johnson, T., Rowland, L. M., Ashraf, M. S., Clark, C. T., Dotson, V. M., Livinski, A. A. & Simon, M.** (2024). Key Findings from Mental Health Research During the Menopause Transition for Racially and Ethnically Minoritized Women Living in the United States: A Scoping Review. *Journal of women's health (2002), 33*(2), 113–131. https://doi.org/10.1089/jwh.2023.0276

• **McKnight, K. K. et al.** (2011). *Racial and regional differences in age at menopause in the United States: findings from the Reasons for Geographic And Racial Differences in Stroke (REGARDS) study. American Journal of Obstetrics and Gynecology, 205*(4), 353.e1–353.e3538. https://doi.org/10.1016/j.ajog.2011.05.014

• **Pershad, A., Morris, J. M., Pace, D. & Khanna, P.** (2022). Racial disparities in menopausal hormone therapy acceptance: a pilot study. *Menopause (New York, N.Y.), 29*(11), 1263–1268. https://doi.org/10.1097/GME.0000000000002061

• **Reeves, A., Elliott, M. R., Karvonen-Gutierrez, C. A. & Harlow, S. D.**

(2023). *Systematic exclusion at study commencement masks earlier menopause for Black women in the Study of Women's Health Across the Nation (SWAN). International Journal of Epidemiology, 52*(5), 1612–1623. https://doi.org/10.1093/ije/dyad085
- **University of Michigan School of Public Health.** (2022, February 23). *25 years of research shows insidious effect of racism on Black women's menopausal transition, health.* https://sph.umich.edu/news/2022posts/insidious-effect-of-racism-on-black-womens-menopausal-transition.html
- **Ussher, J. M., Hawkey, A. J. & Perz, J.** (2019). *'Age of despair', or 'when life starts': Migrant and refugee women negotiate constructions of menopause. Culture, Health & Sexuality, 21*(7), 741–756. https://doi.org/10.1080/13691058.2018.1514069
- **Wallace, B. & Baker, T.** (2025). *Reframing menopause by honouring the lived experiences of Black women. The Lancet Obstetrics, Gynaecology, & Women's Health, 1*(2), e92. https://doi.org/10.1016/j.lanogw.2025.09.002
- **Williams, D. R., Lawrence, J. A. & Davis, B. A.** (2019). *Racism and health: Evidence and needed research. Annual Review of Public Health, 40*, 105–125. https://doi.org/10.1146/annurev-publhealth-040218-043750

10. Indigenous menopause, culture, and health equity

- **Chadha, N., Chadha, V., Ross, S. & Sydora, B. C.** (2016). *Experience of menopause in aboriginal women: A systematic review. Climacteric: The Journal of the International Menopause Society, 19*(1), 17–26. https://doi.org/10.3109/13697137.2015.1119112
- **Gore, M. & Morgan, J.** (2025). *Indigenous women's experiences, symptomology and understandings of menopause: A scoping review. BMC Women's Health, 25*(1), 408. https://doi.org/10.1186/s12905-025-03953-3
- **Kent-Marvick, J. et al.** (2025). *Indigenous, integrative, and biomedical perimenopause and postmenopause healthcare for Indigenous midlife peoples residing in the United States and Canada: A scoping review. medRxiv: The Preprint Server for Health Sciences*, 2025.07.10.25331221. https://doi.org/10.1101/2025.07.10.25331221

11. Policy, public health, inclusive language, workplace, and conceptual framing

- **Davis, S. R., Lambrinoudaki, I. & Lumsden, M. A.** (2023). *Global consensus statement on menopause care and the need for inclusive frameworks. Climacteric, 26*(5), 441–453.
- **Drysdale, K., Creagh, N. S., Nightingale, C., Whop, L. J. & Kelly-Hanku,**

A. (2024). *Inclusive language in health policy – a timely case (study) of cervical screening in Australia. Health Sociology Review, 0*(0), 1–17. https://doi.org/10.1080/14461242.2024.2356868

- **Drysdale, K., Creagh, N. S., Nightingale, C., Whop, L. J. & Kelly-Hanku, A.** (2025). *Beyond words: Operationalizing inclusive language in Australian cervical screening health promotion policy. Health Promotion International, 40*(3), daaf058. https://doi.org/10.1093/heapro/daaf058
- **Garlick, D.** (2024, October 28). *Neurodiversity and menopause: What employers need to know. Menopause in the Workplace.* https://menopauseintheworkplace.co.uk/equality/neurodiversity-and-menopause-what-employers-need-to-know/
- **Guérin, Y., Maguire, F., Clancy, A. & Stairs, J.** (2026). *Beyond "women's" health: A natural language processing analysis of trends in gender-neutral language use. Journal of Obstetrics and Gynaecology Canada, 48*(2), 103199. https://doi.org/10.1016/j.jogc.2025.103199
- **Manion, C. & Shah, S.** (2019). *Decolonizing counseling: Power, privilege, and essentialism in critical feminist practice. Journal of Feminist Family Therapy, 31*(2), 123–141. https://doi.org/10.1080/08952833.2019.1571234
- **Meyer, V. F.** (2001). *The medicalization of menopause: Critique and consequences. International Journal of Health Services, 31*(4), 769–792. https://doi.org/10.2190/m77d-yv2y-d5nu-fxnw
- **Polo-Kantola, P. & Rantala, M. J.** (2019). Menopause, a curse or an opportunity? An evolutionary biological view. *Acta obstetricia et gynecologica Scandinavica, 98*(6), 687–688. https://doi.org/10.1111/aogs.13628
- **Thomas, S. L., Randle, M. & White, S. L.** (2024). *(Re)framing menopause: A comprehensive public health approach. Health Promotion International, 39*(3), daae052. https://doi.org/10.1093/heapro/daae052

* * *

This QR code takes you to a Google doc that houses this bibliography. It's a living document that I will continue to update, so chances are, there may be sources listed in the doc that did not make it into this book. I intend to add new categories as well, as one of my new hyperfocuses is hypermobility.

Afterword

The Next Wave: Research, Advocacy, and a Neurodivergent Peri/Menopause Revolution

Finding yourself stranded at the crossroads of menopause and neurodivergence often means facing a peculiar kind of invisibility. It is not just that the right support is missing; it is that the spaces you turn to for comfort or understanding seem built for someone else entirely. Menopause communities, whether online or in person, tend to center the experiences of cisgender women who seem way less neurocomplex than you. Discussions focus on hot flashes, sleep struggles, and mood swings, but rarely touch on what it is like to have every sense amplified or to lose the ability to organize simple daily routines. Attending a support meeting or reading mainstream advice can feel like eavesdropping on a conversation where your questions do not belong. The expectation is that you "just need to take better care of yourself," as if tracking your cycle on a calendar or meditating each morning solves the confusion that surges when your brain and body refuse to follow any predictable pattern.

On the other hand, neurodivergent forums—spaces built for people with ADHD, autism, or other neurotypes—may not be any more welcoming when it comes to menopause. In these communities, discussions might focus on masking, stimming, or workplace accommodations, but questions about hormone therapy or sudden physical changes are often met with silence or awkward redirection. A search for "menopause" in these forums might return only scattered threads with few replies. For many, this silence rings louder than any outright rejection.

Asking for advice can expose you to the well-worn phrases: "You're too young to be thinking about that," or "Just focus on your ADHD management plan." Even in spaces designed for neurodivergent minds, menopause has been treated as irrelevant, off-topic, or even embarrassing, though, culture is shifting for sure.

The emotional toll of this erasure runs deep. **When you repeatedly encounter advice that fails to address your reality, shame and isolation grow.** Being told to "just exercise more," as if that alone will clear brain fog or tame sensory overload, misses the point entirely. The frustration compounds when friends or family echo the same lines: "You're overthinking it," or "Everyone forgets things at your age." These dismissals sting because they suggest your struggles are either imaginary or self-inflicted. It's like shouting into a void—nobody hears you, nobody even knows what you're asking for. The loneliness becomes acute when neither menopause nor neurodivergence communities offer validation, leaving you with nowhere to set down your burdens.

For those whose identities intersect with race, gender diversity, sexuality, or disability, invisibility multiplies. Black women repeatedly report being dismissed not only by menopause clinics but also by neurodivergent spaces that fail to address how medical bias and cultural stereotypes impact their care. A nonbinary autistic person may enter a "women's health" group hoping for answers and instead encounters language and assumptions that erase their identity. A Latina woman with ADHD navigating menopause may face language barriers, financial limitations, and healthcare providers who rely on stereotypes or offer minimal support. Her experience goes beyond hormonal or executive function: it involves inaccessible forms, rushed appointments without interpreters, misinterpreted symptoms, and limited insurance. If she is also queer or disabled, obstacles increase further. Queer disabled people are often faced with resources that assume financial stability, access to specialists, and family support—privileges not equally distributed.

Add circumstances like cancer survival and/or common co-occurring conditions like PoTS (Postural Orthostatic Tachycardia Syndrome, a blood circulation disorder and a form of dysautonomia — a disorder of the autonomic nervous system), PMDD (Premenstrual Dysphoric Disorder, a severe chronic form of PMS), the connective tissue disorder hEDS (Hypermobile Ehrlers-Danlos Syndrome), endometriosis, MCAS (Mast Cell Activation Syndrome), Hashimoto's disease—and the list goes on and on—and you begin to understand, that these layered exclusions mean that many must translate every piece of advice through the lens of their lived reality, discarding most of it along the way.

I'm still racked with guilt about the fact that I never recorded an audiobook for *The Overthinking Chronicles* when it came out over two years ago, fully aware that this was an accommodation that many folks who followed me on Instagram genuinely needed. Many friends told me that they wanted to read the book but that they were dyslexic like me and/or that one of the significant effects of their ADHD had always included difficulty reading and processing written info. On that note, a beta-reader texted me just after she started reading this book to express her gratitude for the format. She wrote:

> SO grateful you took the ADHD/dyslexia into account when creating this! It's fantastic and really an easy read so far!!! The page where you describe what you did to make it more dyslexic friendly is something that I feel like I would like to share with the world! I think more people need to understand how to make their writing more accessible. It's a game changer for some of us!!!!

Around the same time, a nonbinary reader shared this moving testimony:

> Unlike other books, homepages, or social media accounts about menopause, I haven't been ignored, or treated as an anomaly, or something so disturbing that I can't even be mentioned. *The Neurodivergent Hormonal Survival Toolkit* does not deny my very existence because of the author's 'religion'.

Another nonbinary reader also texted me recently to say "Only on page 36. Have already cried three times," confiding that they wanted "to buy a copy of this book for every ND AFAB person in my life" and that "There aren't words to contain the feeling in my chest of finally being SEEN like this." While this feedback communicates to me that these readers who are so often excluded from spaces feel seen, it paradoxically makes me feel seen in a way I never thought possible, and that's just fucking beautiful. Win-Win.

Here's the thing, though: the last thing I wanted to do was create another well-intended resource that would end up reinforcing this invisibility by centering only "default" stories—those of white, middle-class, cisgender women with access to comprehensive healthcare and supportive families. But the fact is, that is very much the space I get to inhabit for the most part: I know I'm privileged. Nevertheless, I still reached a point where I felt like I was left to navigate menopause with an ND brain alone and unseen, forced to become an expert in my own body because nobody else was going to do it for me. I knew if I felt this way that it was most certainly exponentially worse for BIPOC communities and gender-expansive, nonbinary and trans folks. The pain of exclusion does not just come from ignorance; it comes from being erased by omission, and I don't want anyone to experience this.

* * *

It's now 2026. Social media is starting to overflow with wellness influencers, therapists, coaches, medical providers, and, haha, yes, advocates like myself offering advice on menopause, guides promising relief from hot flashes and mood swings, supplements, the next trending solution to your "problems." But for a long time, the majority rarely discussed sensory overload or executive dysfunction. While we have seen a shift in just the past year with some attention finally being given to the intersection of neurodivergence and hormonal fluctuations, many of these new books, guides, and published studies still don't acknowledge the complexity of neurodivergence, and it starts to seem like the term 'neurodivergent' is being reduced to just ADHD and/or Autism.

This book exists to play a role in bridging these gaps. My aim was not empty reassurance, but practical strategies, research-backed facts, and stories that hopefully reflect some of your reality. I hope you were able to find anecdotes that echo your confusion, and guidance for when clarity emerges. Learning to decode which symptoms are hormonal, which are tied to your neurotype, and—most crucially—what you can actually do about them is challenging and takes time, a keen sense of self awareness, and perhaps even some arduous trial and error with a variety of treatments.

I called this book a survival toolkit because it is a lifeline, not just a reference guide, and one that I so desperately needed 5-10 years ago. I have read stacks of peer-reviewed studies, listened to hundreds of stories, responded to possibly thousands of DMs on social media at this point, created the ADHD Peri Punks Podcast and community with my co-host, Chrissy Ingram, facilitated an expert panel on hormones and neurodivergence at the NeuroDiversion event in Austin, Texas in March 2026, and gathered and created the best tools I could conceptualize. I hope this book helps you cut through confusion and find clarity. You will not have to guess which information is trustworthy, or which strategies work for brains like ours.

My ultimate goal was to have this book be a resource that does not perpetuate erasure. It is far from perfect or exhaustive, nor will it be embraced enthusiastically by everyone. And that's ok. No one is for everyone, and the impact it's already had on early readers and reviewers has legit blown my mind. I am honored to be a part of any work that promotes inclusion with real impact, not just good intentions, and in that sense, I hope that this mission was accomplished for you as well. I don't take for granted that you have a choice in terms of whom you trust and how you spend your money. The fact that you chose to buy this book is not lost on me, and I thank you.

The reality remains, however, that a) I am not a clinician or medical provider, and b) I am a white, privileged cis woman, and c) as I just said, most menopause research still centers on "neurotypical" women. Clinical trials, academic studies, and surveys often neglect the realities of neurodivergent adults, and the ones that do treat neurodivergence often focus on just ADHD and Autism and thus, more complex and nuanced ND experiences go largely unrecognized.

So what can we do? We advocate first and foremost for ourselves— because self-care is community care—and then we start advocating for the collective.

Intersectional advocacy recognizes how overlapping identities—race, class, gender, disability, neurotype—create unique barriers in midlife care and support. Addressing menopause or neurodivergence in isolation is insufficient; these challenges compound when they intersect. Intersectional advocacy means acknowledging these complexities, not oversimplifying them.

Practical strategies can open doors in healthcare.

Collaborate with allies—patients, clinicians, or advocates—especially those who grasp the complexity of neurodivergent menopause. Co-advocacy, even online, amplifies your voice.

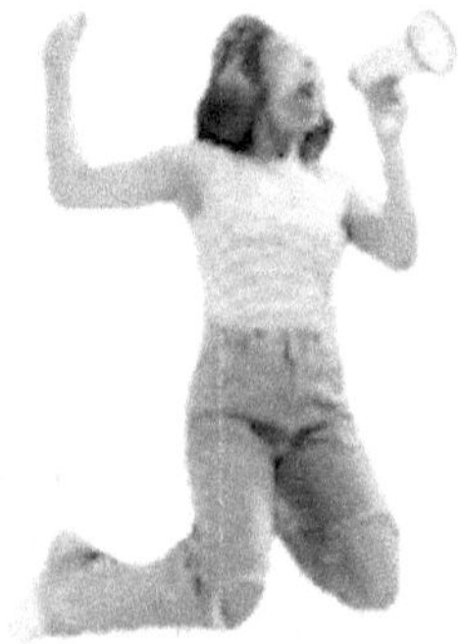

File complaints as a means for change, not just for emergencies. Provide specific feedback, such as, "During my last appointment, I was not offered translation services, and my sensory needs were ignored. This impacted my care."

Use patient feedback forms or adapt a template:

"Dear [Clinic/Hospital Name], I am writing to share my experience as a neurodivergent patient in menopause. My care was affected by [describe issue]. I recommend [solution—language access, sensory-friendly spaces, staff training]. Thank you for considering this."

Joining or creating a patient advisory board gives you influence over clinic policies and practices, and these boards often seek underrepresented voices—your lived experience is valuable here.

Broad, systemic changes emerge when more voices join together. Patient advisory boards can advocate for things like sensory-friendly appointment slots, multilingual information, and neuroaffirming staff training. If your clinic lacks such a board, inquire about starting one focused on neurodiversity and menopause. Present local survey results or research that highlight care gaps, and invite staff and patients to suggest needed changes.

This is how we start to shift the narrative and the literal evidence.

Your perspective is essential—there are gaps only your voice and others like yours can fill. By sharing your story, you help shape the future of care, policy, and understanding, rewriting what's possible for neurodivergent people in midlife.

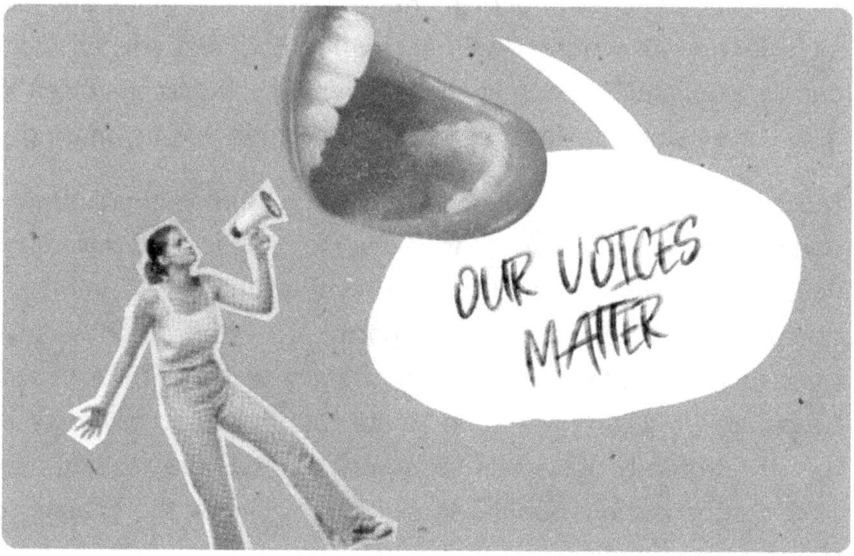

Getting involved in research studies is easier than you might think. Many studies now actively seek neurodivergent midlife participants. Universities are increasingly working with patient advisors, gathering both structured data and personal testimonials. Frequently, you can participate through online forms or calls for contributors on research and advocacy websites.

You don't have to wait for an invitation. Start by gathering your thoughts on significant moments and experiences. A story template might look like:

"My name is/my pronouns are [first name or pseudonym]. I am [your age], [your neurotype(s)], and I am experiencing [perimenopause/menopause]. My biggest challenge has been [describe]. One thing that helped me was [describe]. I wish providers/partners/friends understood [describe]."

You can submit these to research teams, nonprofits, or surveys —often anonymously. Bullet points or audio recordings are just as effective if writing feels overwhelming. Patient advisory panels also value authentic stories and recruit diverse voices to help shape study designs, surveys, and identify what's missing.

Inclusive research teams actively welcome neurodivergent perspectives, prioritizing gender-diverse, BIPOC, and late-diagnosed participants. Look for universities known for intersectional health research or teams partnered with neurodiversity-focused organizations. Researchers such as **Dr. Aimee Grant**, Associate Professor of Public Health at Swansea University in the UK, regularly post calls for contributors. Some studies may offer compensation, public recognition, or simply the chance to shape understanding.

Dr. Grant currently has a research project called **Autism Menstruation to Menopause**, a study that "aims to create new understandings of reproductive health experiences of Autistic women and others with wombs across the lifecourse," which "includes things like periods, contraception, endometriosis and other gynaecological conditions, and menopause."

Led by a community council with diverse, intersecting identities, the project focuses on the impact of racism, classism, and anti-LGBTQ+ bias on healthcare experiences. The website (autism menstruationtomenopause.com) points out that the project "is Autistic-led and is co-governed by a Community Council of Autistic people," noting that they have recently begun contacting participants, which "will involve 100 Autistic people taking part in 10 interviews each over a 5-year period." The project has been ongoing for several years now and ends in October 2030, with the goal being "to design tools to make healthcare more accessible for Autistic people." It's been intentionally designed to center marginalized voices, actively seeking diverse samples across race, ethnicity, and gender identity.

Ultimately, **advocacy strengthens when more people join.** Even if you don't consider yourself an "advocate," you can mentor someone just diagnosed or support a peer through their first hot flash or doctor's appointment. You can host a panel or webinar with a few participants on topics such as "ADHD and menopause at work" or "Sensory-friendly self-care in midlife." Libraries, community centers, and online platforms can facilitate these events. Promoting these resources, even with a simple flyer or post, helps connect those seeking help.

Mentorship doesn't require expertise, just honesty and willingness to help.

You might guide someone in writing a doctor's letter, demystifying symptom trackers, or simply sharing what worked—or didn't—for you. Awareness efforts can also include writing to local papers, creating educational social media posts, or joining national awareness campaigns around neurodiversity and menopause. Even a single social post can ignite a needed conversation.

Imagine a future where **intersectional inclusive neurodivergent menopause** is acknowledged as a legitimate life stage: clinics use inclusive forms, workplaces automatically offer sensory-friendly options, and resources address every kind of body and mind. Researchers proactively seek neurodivergent perspectives. When you share your truth, you clear the way for future generations. We are at a tipping point; your contribution helps drive this cultural shift.

This vision is steadily becoming reality, built by those who speak up. The future can be inclusive and neuroaffirming, filled with possibility. Every shared story strengthens this movement.

In summary, your experience provides answers that research seeks, advocacy needs, and future generations will rely on.

Whether you participate in studies, lead projects, or help just one other person through a hard day, you are shaping a world that recognizes and supports every neurocomplex person in midlife.

Acknowledgements

AKA It Takes a Village...

Short story long...

I am so grateful for **my family, my siblings, my kids, and especially my partner, John,** who is genuinely my biggest fan and greatest admirer. He believes in me like no one ever has and doesn't bat an eye each time I unveil my latest diabolically "hare-brained" scheme to create a passive income stream that will simultaneously save the planet and allow me to be the most generous benefactor to the arts/prolific world traveler.

And of course, **to my life-long friends.** You know who you are. We may not have known I was ADHD until very recently, but I know y'all inherently understand that when I get hyperfocused on something, you'll be stuck listening to me talk about it until I'm done talking about it. Thanks for putting up with me creating a new Instagram account where I subsequently made a ton of new friends revolving around this recent life pivot for me, and then, due to limited capacity, pretty much abandoned posting on my personal IG and Facebook. You all have known me longer than anyone, and I will always love you. Thank you for loving me, too, no matter what.

* * *

But, let's get down to brass tacks: a whole is only as good as the sum of its parts. I appreciate the village it takes to have projects like this come to fruition. Here are my villagers:

Thank you to my newest friends and partners in this work, co-founders of **The NeuroPause Collective:**

Meredith Carder, Mandi Dixon, Sera Gray, Chrissy Ingram, Kristin Koliha, Julie Murillas, and Jen Wolkin. This book is better because of the countless one-on-one conversations I've had with each of you, as well as the ones that included all of us collectively. Thanks to each of you for your individual contributions to this book. Early readers are so important, and I don't underestimate the gift I was given by having seven credentialed ND peri/menopausal women with "bonus" lived experience read a draft. Your editorial blurbs are a crucial highlight, and Mandi, the beautiful foreword you so generously penned with zero hesitation captures just what I hoped to communicate: how real and unpretentious both you and I are as people, and ultimately, thus, this book as well. I'm so grateful that the stars aligned as they did and brought the eight of us together (literally, too, since we've all met in real life now) in the passionate pursuit of this mission driven work to advocate for intersectional neuroinclusivity and hormonal justice. Your professional expertises coupled with your raw humor and humanity enrich my life daily, and I fucking love y'all.

Thank you to **Hédi Assmann and Kristen Maple** for their proofreading prowess. Proofreading and editing are crucial in the writing and publishing process, and they found major errors that even surprised my eagle eyes!

A heartfelt thank you, also, to **Vanessa Weiland**, who offered fantastic critical feedback as a prescribing provider specializing in menopause care. Her medical expertise helped me learn new things, make important content adjustments, and even a couple additions to this book.

Thanks to all who took the time to read an advance copy and provide such thoughtful and impactful reviews and testimonials, which genuinely play a significant part in the marketing and potential reach of books. If you skipped the "Praise for" section at the very beginning, go check it out to see all the names, credentials, and words of the specialists who felt this book was good enough to associate their name with! They humble me.

When it comes down to it, though, there are two people, especially, who are indisputably responsible for the sheer existence of this book and its eventual evolution into what you hold in your hands.

Firstly, this book would have never existed had I never met **Chrissy Ingram**, my New Zealander punk sister currently living in the Australian Outback, and that is the cold hard truth. I first met Chrissy Online in 2022 from an IG account I had on punk. We became friends over the course of several months, leaving messages for each other in the DMs on Instagram. But it was that fateful day in June 2023 that changed everything. I remember it very clearly. We had recently decided to start communicating via WhatsApp, leaving each other podcast-length voice notes. One day, I hit her up with an enthusiasm I hadn't felt in ages. "Chrissy!" I said. "You should totally do a podcast with me on mental health!"

She countered, almost immediately with this: "How about you do a podcast with me on ADHD and perimenopause?"

So specific, haha. So niche. I didn't even have my ADHD diagnosis yet, and I didn't know shit about perimenopause, despite the fact that it had been rocking my world adversely for the previous decade, but I didn't hesitate. My answer was an instantaneous "fuck yes, let's go," and the rest is history. That is THE reason this book exists. This was the turning point that gave me new direction and purpose in life, and I had no idea how deep it was going to get, nor the rollercoaster I'd be riding to reach the place I am as I write this.

But it's not just the existence of the book. I also have to thank **Chrissy** for reading the very first completed draft in the summer of 2025. She provided crucial notes regarding format, the visuals, and the overall accessibility of the information, as well as feedback about the urgency around the suicidal ideation that can occur as a result of hormonal havoc colliding with neurodivergent brains. It's those initial conversations with Chrissy that spawned the more intentional format of the book and all the design decisions that make it more accessible for ND brains: from font style and size, letter and line spacing, and uniform structure, to lighter info density and varied presentations of info blocks, and the deliberate choice to intermittently integrate images throughout.

And finally, I would be remiss (and frankly, delusional lol), however, to not thank **Lasara Firefox Allen** for the pivotal role they played in the intentional reframing of so much of the language of the book. Reading Lasara's own revolutionary book *Genderqueer Menopause* and completing their certification course on Gender Affirming Menopause Care made me suspect that my book still needed a lot of work. I decided to postpone the launch and do a full audit for more inclusive language, and it was a disconcerting revelation. I realized that despite what I had believed to be the solidly inclusive ethos of the book, much of the language was still rooted strongly in a gender binary throughout and in essence, therefore, not very inclusive at all. The horror! In the end, this language shift inevitably led to some changes in concrete content as well, resulting in the book you hold now.

I hope I'm not forgetting anyone. Unfortunately, forgetfulness is a hallmark of both ADHD and peri/menopause, so please don't RSD your ass off if you helped me majorly and were not mentioned. I swear I appreciate you.

Recommended Reads

Carder, Meredith. *It All Makes Sense Now: Embrace Your ADHD Brain to Live a Creative and Colorful Life.* Hay House, 2024.

Meredith writes like someone who actually gets what it feels like to live inside an ADHD brain without flattening it into a meme or a motivational poster. Because she's the real deal and also a friend, I can say with my full chest that this book is warm, useful, and wildly affirming without ever talking down to the reader. Bonus: She also talks a bit about hormones in it.

Conner, Alex, and James Brown. *ADHD Unpacked: The Ultimate Guide to Understanding Your Adult ADHD from the Hosts of The ADHD Adults Podcast.* Bloomsbury Publishing, 2025.

This one has the rare gift of being both grounded in science and readable by people whose brains would rather sprint naked through traffic than finish a dense self-help book. It's clear, funny, unsnobby, and actually useful, which is a miracle genre combo.

Corinna, Heather. *What Fresh Hell Is This? Perimenopause, Menopause, Other Indignities, and You.* Balance, 2021.

If menopause books have too often sounded like they were written by a scented candle in a cardigan, this one comes in with better timing and sharper teeth. Heather Corinna makes room for rage, absurdity, and bodily chaos without sacrificing compassion or substance. This is menopause with smart (ass) humor and a punk honesty that makes you feel less alone in the chaos.

Eltahawy, Mona, editor. *Bloody Hell!: Adventures in Menopause From Around the World.* Unbound, 2025.

This anthology feels like menopause finally escaped the beige prison of respectability politics and started telling the truth with a multicultural megaphone. It's global, unruly, smart, and gloriously unwilling to behave, which is exactly what the subject deserves. It offers a powerful, broader and more rebellious glimpse of menopause than mainstream books will ever show.

Firefox Allen, Lasara. *Genderqueer Menopause: Navigating Menopause for Trans, Gender-Nonconforming, Genderfluid, and Other Queer-Bodied Folx.* North Atlantic Books, 2026.

This book doesn't just widen the frame; it takes a crowbar to the whole lazy, cis-normative menopause script and rebuilds it with care, precision, and actual humanity. Lasara's work helped me make my own toolkit more inclusive, more accurate, and less likely to accidentally reproduce the same old exclusionary bullshit, and I will be eternally grateful to them for that. Lasara also offers a certification course in gender affirming menopause care. I took it. I loved it. I highly recommend it.

Gunter, Jen. *The Menopause Manifesto: Own Your Health with Facts and Feminism.* Citadel Press, 2021.

Yeah, Dr. Jen Gunter can be polarizing, but she is relentless about evidence, and frankly, you can't blame a bitch for that. This was the first menopause book I read, back when I still didn't know shit about hormones or my own neurodivergent wiring, and it gave me a foundation that was rooted in science and political AF. Everyone loves to hate her now, but her book was my intro into this world, the gateway, and I learned a lot.

Kahn, Gilly. *Allow Me to Interrupt: A Psychologist Reveals the Emotional Truth Behind Women's ADHD.* Post Hill Press, 2025.

Dr. Kahn, AKA Gilly, is a friend, and I'm one of the de-identified women whose lived experience helped inform the research orbit of her book, so yes, you are absolutely welcome to play a deranged little game of "guess which one is Sarah." Friendship bias aside, this book is razor-sharp, clinically grounded, deeply validating about the emotional wreckage and brilliance of women's ADHD, and also creatively written with compelling stories sprinkled with humor and humanity.

Mosconi, Lisa. *The Menopause Brain: New Science Empowers Women to Navigate the Pivotal Transition with Knowledge and Confidence.* Avery, 2024.

This is the book for anyone who wants raw data on brain fog instead of being told they're hysterical and sent to be burned at the stake. Dr. Mosconi takes the neurological side of menopause seriously and gives it the intellectual weight medicine should have given it decades ago.

Nerenberg, Jenara. *Divergent Mind: Thriving in a World That Wasn't Designed for You.* HarperOne, 2021.

This is one of those books that makes a whole population of readers go, "Oh, hell, so that's what has been happening to me." Nerenberg doesn't just describe divergence; she challenges the rotten architecture of normalcy itself, which is frankly a public service. I fucking love this book, and I have read it twice, no small feat for my ADHD dyslexic ass.

Pink, Richard, and Roxanne Emery. *Dirty Laundry: Why Adults with ADHD Are So Ashamed and What We Can Do to Help*. Ten Speed Press, 2023.

This book is especially strong on the emotional fallout of ADHD, particularly shame, self-blame, and relational strain. It is compassionate without becoming syrupy and honest without turning ADHD into misery porn, which gives it unusual credibility and heart.

Rolston, Yansie, and Yvonne Christie, editors. *Black and Menopausal: Intimate Stories of Navigating the Change*. Jessica Kingsley Publishers, 2023.

I love these stories, and every single one offers a compelling and unique perspective. This collection matters because menopause discourse has too often been filtered through whiteness, and that distortion has consequences. By centering Black voices and lived experience, the anthology offers a necessary corrective to the mainstream conversation and expands what menopause literature can and should be.

Walker, Nick. *Neuroqueer Heresies: Notes on the Neurodiversity Paradigm, Autistic Empowerment, and Postnormal Possibilities*. Autonomous Press, 2021.

This is not a beginner-friendly, hand-holding little pamphlet for people who want their paradigm shifts pre-softened. It is theory-rich, liberating, and intellectually fierce, making it a vital text for anyone serious about neurodiversity, queerness, power, and the politics of who gets called disordered.

Wolkin, Jennifer R. *Quick Calm: Easy Meditations to Short-Circuit Stress Using Mindfulness and Neuroscience.* New Harbinger Publications, 2021.

Dr. Jen is SUCH a badass, and I can't recommend this resource enough. This book offers practical tools for nervous-system regulation without drifting into the kind of vague, precious wellness bullshit that makes many readers want to set shit on fire. While multiple resources on anxiety reduction I've tried are steeped in the kind of toxic positivity that legit did the opposite and almost made an arsonist of me, *Quick Calm* is accessible, smart, and deeply respectful of what it actually feels like to live in an overstimulated, overwhelmed brain and body. No need for an extinguisher or a bucket of water. The tears of joy you'll cry from feeling seen will transform the chaotic rage-fueled fires in your brain into the 3-wick lavender candle your soul's been seeking for ages now.

Yuknavitch, Lidia, editor. *The Big M: 13 Writers Take Back the Story of Menopause*. Grand Central Publishing, 2026.

This anthology promises the kind of menopause storytelling that refuses tidy packaging and easy platitudes. Not unlike *Black and Menopausal*, it is compelling precisely because it offers multiple voices and perspectives, pushing back against the idea that there is one respectable or acceptable way to experience this transition.

About the Author

Dr. Sarah L. Glasco (she/her) is a late-diagnosed dyslexic ADHD/OCD writer with hypermobility, IOATH certified gender-affirming menopause care consultant, neurodiversity activist leading clinician outreach for the NeuroDiversion event, and producer, editor & co-host of the ADHD Peri Punks Podcast. She currently spends a significant amount of time trying to drag conversations about neurodivergence, hormones, accessibility, and healthcare equity out of the dark ages.

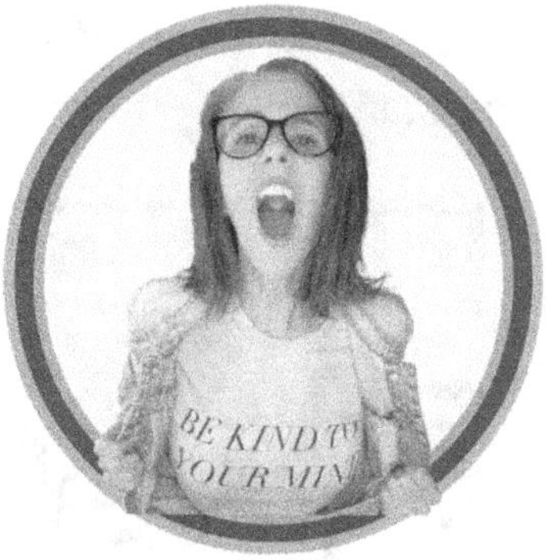

A former tenured college professor, published scholar, classically trained 'cellist, multi-instrumentalist rock musician, and mom to two adult neurodivergent kids, Sarah has lived and worked in both the UK and France. She has most recently presented research on neuroinclusive teaching and learning at the International ADHD Conference in 2025 and facilitated an expert panel on the intersection of hormones and neurodivergence at NeuroDiversion in March 2026.

Her work focuses on the frequently ignored intersection of neurodivergence, hormones, burnout, identity, accessibility, and systemic inequity, particularly as they affect AFAB and gender-expansive people navigating peri/menopause and beyond. She is especially interested in the ways capitalism, patriarchy, medical misogyny, ableism, and chronic masking quietly grind neurodivergent people into dust while still expecting them to answer emails professionally.

Her current hyper-fixations include neurodivergence & AFAB people's health, hyping her people up, smashing patriarchy rooted in white supremacy, a good night's sleep, and living life on her own terms. Otherwise, she fancies herself a free-lance existentialist philosopher, purveyor of dark sarcasm, and lead clown of her own circus.

Also by Sarah L. Glasco, PhD

-*The Overthinking Chronicles: Cultivating Your Inner Comedian to Reframe Anxiety, Spark Self-Compassion and Trust, and Give Self-Doubt the Punchline It Deserves* (Mod Couple Press, 2024) [Published under the pen name Sara Toninstan]

As well as this lit-crit gem from her academic life:

-*Parody and Palimpsest: Intertextuality, Language and the Ludic in the Novels of Jean-Philippe Toussaint.* New York, Peter Lang, 2015.

For the extra-curious and downright nosey, you can find a list of academic publications from her previous life as a professor by scanning the QR code. ➡➡➡ .

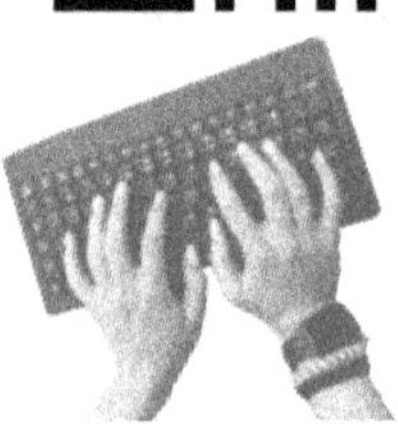

You can also find her essays on SubStack at @sarcrassticselfcare and @adhdperipunks.

She tends to intermittently rant and lurk on Instagram as well at @sarcrasstic.self.care, @adhdperipunks + @neuropausecollective.

www.ingramcontent.com/pod-product-compliance
Lightning Source LLC
LaVergne TN
LVHW022159200926
848481LV00006B/1786